Glass House Books
4 Pillars: Creating a Life on YOUR Terms

Geoff Smith is a student of yoga, rugby coach, personal trainer and teacher with over 20 years' experience. He holds a Master of Education, an MBA and post graduate certificates in management and leadership. In his role as an educational leader in schools for at-risk youth, Geoff introduces the principles of the 4 Pillars to manage burnout among fellow staff and to create enhanced levels of wellbeing and excellence. Geoff lives in Brisbane, Australia with his fiancé Ash and dog Bodhi.

I0027270

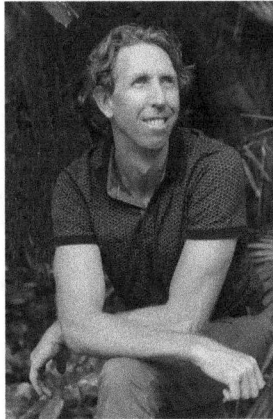

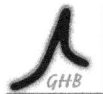

Glass House Books
Brisbane

Glass House Books
an imprint of IP (Interactive Publications Pty Ltd)
Treetop Studio • 9 Kuhler Court
Carindale, Queensland, Australia 4152
sales@ipoz.biz
http://ipoz.biz/

Printed in 12 pt Adobe Caslon Pro on 14 pt Avenir Book.

ISBN: 9781922830005 (PB); 9781922830012 (eBk)

A catalogue record for this book is available from the National Library of Australia

Project Kindy

A percentage of copies sold will be donated to support this charity.
Website https://projectkindy.com/

4 Pillars:
Creating a Life
on YOUR Terms

Geoff Smith

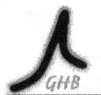

Glass House Books
Brisbane

Dedicated to my relationships that inspire, challenge and motivate me to be a better person. My family, my friends and my loving partner, Ash.

Contents

Introduction

Monday morning 3 a.m.

Stillness and silence.

My brother once said that only misfits and those living on the edges of society are awake at this hour. I like the sound of that. Being a misfit has real advantages.

Early morning is the time for writers, innovators, philosophers and artists. It's time to prepare for the day ahead and begin another day investing in the 4 Pillars. These pillars of health, relationships, finance and mindset form the foundation of creating a life on our terms: a life where I now decide how, with whom and where I spend my time. It's how I create a life I define as a success.

It all happens in the early hours while most are asleep. It occurs through preparation and planning. Creating a successful life means becoming uncommon. Rising early was just one of many uncommon traits shared throughout this book.

The 4 Pillars contains the rituals and habits to create a life on your terms. This book also includes strategies to overcome challenges I encountered as I progressed, in an effort to share an authentic account of personal development and improvement. Tough times often reveal more about our inadequacies than we like to admit, but they are valuable teachers. Working through each of the 4 pillars and the strategies I use to keep moving forward provides a template for choosing your own path as you create a life on your own terms.

Maybe you're faced with adversity right now—adversity in the form of an unsatisfying job, an unfulfilling relationship or a sense of overall fatigue. This book provides strategies based on science, ancient wisdom and personal experience that go beyond exercise programs to flatten your stomach.

The 4 Pillars focuses on unpacking the underlying beliefs and habits currently represented in the life you are living: beliefs and habits that no longer serve the person you are choosing to become.

Together we will explore how to develop habits and rituals that will enhance your performance in all areas of life. We'll also anticipate and investigate challenges that you may encounter in relationships, finances and your mindset that have the potential to sabotage your efforts.

Finally, this book represents the never-ending journey of self-development all of us are taking. There is no finish line. There are no winners or losers. Yet, there is an ocean of fulfilment that unfolds once we seek to become better versions of ourselves.

Regardless of where you are on your journey, this book will provide practical, simple and effective strategies to create the life you desire.

PART I – The Pillars

The secret of change is to focus all of your energy not on fighting the old, but on building the new.
– Socrates

Chapter 1 – Pillar 1: Unshakeable Health

Like any new journey, our initial steps set the course for our destination. There is no time to waste. The 4 PILLARS shows us precisely how to take control of the specific areas in our live that have the greatest impact on our happiness.

Our health is our most important asset. It serves us throughout our entire life. With the right time and attention, we can appreciate the gift of our health, learn the way it communicates to us and develop the right steps to maintain it.

Recently, I was reminded of how the body communicates. I woke up at 12.30a.m. and couldn't get back to sleep. I felt stress building in the center of my chest for the day ahead and listened for the deeper message my body was sending me.

Although I knew I needed to do something about my job before it impacted my health, I had spent the entire weekend working towards solutions. At 12.30a.m. that Monday, the anxiety was there, keeping me awake.

I had two choices: get up and do something or try to sleep it off. I knew from past experience that sleeping it off wasn't going to happen, so I got out of bed. I listened to a yoga nidra meditation for 15 minutes, focused my mind on the challenges at work, and then went back to bed. Within a few minutes, I was asleep. When my alarm went off in the morning, although still tired, I knew I had looked after myself and was in a better frame of mind.

While there are still times when I fail to listen to my body, applying simple techniques affords more control over situations like these. Obtaining knowledge is one thing; knowing when to act on that knowledge is wisdom. That is what the HEALTH PILLAR is all about.

The HEALTH PILLAR includes everything we need to exercise, nourish and recover so we can be at our absolute peak physical condition each day. We wake up each morning prepared for the challenges ahead and satisfied we are doing everything possible to feel our best. We take responsibility to feel unshakeable when the world around us begins to crumble.

Feeling unshakeable is more than being free from disease. Unshakeable health means being prepared for physical challenges throughout the day and navigating through life requires a reservoir of vitality. Unshakeable health is an expression of the energy that enables us to finish the day as well as we began. People with this energy are magnets for great opportunities. They create this energy through their choices, their mindset, and through the circumstances around them.

The Health Pillar also includes the presentation of our body to the world. Presentation is the clothes we choose to wear, the effort we put into our appearance, and the care we give to our physical form. It's our body language and engagement when meeting a person for the first time and the decisions we make around what food to eat at the end of a challenging day.

Our primary care to ourselves is the basis for providing care to others. We cannot give what we don't have and taking care of our physical health is the first step in authentically helping those around us.

The total health care championed in this book does not come naturally for many people. Our task is to take responsibility and prioritize our wellbeing even with people in our lives who depend on us. Throughout this book, we'll explore how many small, consistent changes lead to significant progress.

Total health care reminds us that the harder we are on something, the faster we wear it out. This principle applies in how we drive our cars, enjoy our intimate relationships and how we care for ourselves. In relation to health, the harder we punish ourselves through excessive eating or extreme and punishing exercise regimes, the earlier we will see signs of wear and tear. Visible through aches and pains, injuries or a growing waistline. Even small actions of care can have large impacts on health, wellbeing and vitality.

There Are No Shortcuts

There are no shortcuts in developing and maintaining optimal health. Like many people, I have looked for shortcuts and easy answers when there weren't any. Short cuts like popular dieting trends or fad exercise routines resulting in inconsistent results. The health pillar invites us to appreciate that there are no shortcuts in developing unshakeable health.

Now is the time to eradicate the mindset that looks for easy answers for our health. Answers that we have outsourced to third parties. Now is the time to become the expert on YOUR health. To understand and appreciate your body, how it functions and what it requires to be at its best.

This is particularly important as we age. In our youth, we can take our health for granted and get away with it. We can endure the late nights, the poor eating habits and the substance abuse that comes from excess. However, as we age, the consequences for this mistreatment can accumulate. Untreated sporting injuries, a growing waistline or lack of vitality are all symptoms of a body in need of assistance. The health pillar is our foundation for regaining control with our life.

Who says that as we age, we cannot enjoy remarkable health and vitality? Society may push the story of depletion and disease as we age but I am sure we all know people who maintain vibrancy well into their 80's, 90's and beyond!

Focusing on the health pillar allows us to appreciate how progress in one area has the potential to influence the remaining pillars. It's easy to think that each pillar operates in its own silo. However, each pillar is interrelated. Improvement of one pillar can substantially enhance and stabilize the performance of the others.

For example, if we are feeling good about our physical appearance, feeling physically strong and fit, and presenting ourselves at our best through the food we eat and the clothes we wear, our mindset will be strong and positive. From this place, we feel good about our relationships and have the confidence to take positive action in those relationships, leading to enhanced self-worth and happiness. Once we see our work into action, it becomes addictive, pulling us further forward.

Defining Health Success

Discard the perception of obtaining the perfect body. Perfection in anything is a state of mind and only sets us up for failure. Remember, the body includes not only our physical health and wellbeing but also our nutrition, sleep and presentation. Our body is constantly changing and by comparing our physical body to others will only lead to self-judgement and a negative mindset. Understanding what our body requires allows us to make more informed decisions along a path toward unshakeable health.

Take sleep, for example. How much sleep do we need each night to wake up feeling refreshed and energized? For some people, it may mean only five to six hours. For others, it might be substantially more. The exact number of hours isn't as important as getting a feel for what we need in order to be at our best. Some days, too, we need more sleep than others and that's fine. Over time, developing an understanding of our requirements allows us to determine when we need to be in bed to function at our best. Knowing the impact of not getting enough sleep and how it affects our performance also assists us in determining our sleep patterns. Some people are early risers and are more productive early in the morning, while others function better in the evening. Experiment with what works for you until you have a baseline. We know intuitively what our body needs and creating structure and habits to support our requirements helps us stay on track.

Nutrition is another example of contradictory information. High or low fat, high protein, low carbohydrates, and other confusing recommendations have come and gone over the last 50 years and can overwhelm our best intentions. Everyone has a different body that requires a different nutrient approach and what may work for one person may not work for others. Our bodies and our nutritional needs are constantly changing, so just because we ate a particular way in the past, does not necessarily mean that it still serves our needs today.

Read that passage again. Are we attached to a diet or pattern of thinking that may have worked for us in the past and no longer serves our needs today? To create a life on our terms, are we open to surrender old habits, routines and even foods that were once important for us?

There have been times when I have loved a meal so much that I thought I would be eating it for the rest of my life. A particular type of breakfast would satisfy my needs so much that I would envisage consuming it for the rest of my life. However, as I have gotten older, new foods and combinations have come up on my 'must have' list. All exemplifying our ever-changing nutritional needs. Consciously exploring and observing the impact different food has on our energy levels, our productivity and fluctuations in our emotions can empower us to make healthy adaptations as we age.

We are living examples of the food we eat. What we put into our mouths becomes who we are. Dr. Alberto Villoldo, in *Grow a New Body* (2019) insists that with the right combination of nutrition and food, we can not only heal ourselves physically but also spiritually transform our being. As a psychologist and medical anthropologist, he investigates how food impacts our psychological mindset and our ability to overcome challenges we face. With this new-found awareness, we can literally choose to become the version of ourselves we hope to become.

The food we eat not only provides fuel for our bodies, but also meets many of our emotional needs. Understanding the link between nutrition and emotions can enable us to see patterns of behaviour and associated eating during times of stress. Perhaps, when faced with challenges, we instinctively turn to food for comfort while avoiding our actual problem. While enjoying our favorite food is part of life, we know problems arise when those foods control us and become an addiction.

We might also unconsciously sabotage our efforts for self-development through an addictive habit with food, poor nutrition and lack of hydration. A large percentage of our bodies and cells are composed of water and according to H. Mitchell in the *Journal of Biological Chemistry 158*, vital organs such as the brain, heart, lungs and skin all require considerable and constant hydration. Drinking an adequate amount of water each day is a simple and effective way to improve our health. Creating habits of drinking purified water or taking water to work each day, allows us to control the quality and quantity of what we consume. Purchasing a high-quality water filter and water bottle is a relatively small investment in our health.

How we present ourselves to the world is a dimension of the body with great implications on our mindset. Our presentation and the time we take in presenting ourselves at our best sends clear messages to those around us as to who we believe we are. Taking the time to present ourselves is not about purchasing the best clothes or wearing the most expensive accessories. Our presentation is an attitude towards ourselves and what we have to offer. We develop a belief that we expect great things to happen, and it is reflected in our posture, our facial expressions and our body language. We are open to the world and position ourselves to receive the very best of it.

This can be challenging work. Self-judgement, comparison and negative self-talk can sabotage our efforts. Other people, particularly friends and colleagues, may feel threatened by our efforts and criticize us. It's OK to 'fake it until you make it' to move beyond any resistance. Remember, our presentation is about opening up to the world that we are destined for bigger and better things. Sometimes we have to 'act' in a certain role until we become comfortable in it.

The final dimension of the health pillar to consider is our breath. We know that without it, we can only last a matter of minutes before we die. Without a sufficient range of breathing our quality of life diminishes and illness can easily take hold. Devoting time to improve the quality, depth and capacity of our breathing is an essential element in our health and in taking on the challenges we set ourselves. We can control our breath in times of crisis and use it to purify the body and mind.

Sleep, fitness, nutrition, water-intake, presentation and breathwork are a few of the areas we must consider for thriving health. It is our responsibility to keep it operating at its peak.

Success within the body dimension of the 4 Pillars means that we schedule our day to create habits and routines that support the continual maintenance and growth of this incredible gift. Optimizing these dimensions of health and working on each of them daily offers amazing results over a short period of time. The impact of this optimization will also quickly cascade into the remaining 3 Pillars, positively impacting on them as well.

Summary

Total health care is rare. Energy and vitality are necessary to create a life on our terms. Energy is everything. It is the invisible force that will enable us to develop momentum and push through challengers. The energy we receive through our exercise regime, the food we consume, the fluids we drink and the quality of our sleep will influence every area of our life. The decisions we make regarding our health reverberate in our relationships, finances and our mindset.

The investment of time, energy and resources we give to our bodies is a foundation for the 4 Pillars. We acquire insights and knowledge and take action to present our bodies at their best. We develop unshakeable health that enables us to move through each day with energy and vitality. The investment we make in our body has the potential to improve our physical health and wellbeing and also positively impact the remaining 3 Pillars.

Reflections

No one else can enter our thoughts and determine where we are in life and how close we are to our goals. Often, we gather our perspectives and beliefs about ourselves from the outside world and rarely take time to ask the deeper questions. These chapter reflections are designed to shift our attention inwards to the person we are and the person we desire to become.

Ask yourself, are you currently living your best life?

Be honest.

It may appear differently to the outside world, and it may appear that you are achieving in all areas, and yet you may sense imbalance or a lack of fulfilment.

Spend no more than a few minutes on each activity and write out a couple of sentences as to why you have given that answer. These reflections develop a new sense of awareness within you that will ultimately lead to small but significant changes over a long period of time.

Activities

1. Reflect on the Health Pillars and give yourself a rating of 1–10 for each category, with 10 being ideal.

   - Physical health
   - Energy levels throughout the day
   - Effort in appearance
   - Sleep
   - Nutritional intake

2. What does great health and vitality mean for you?

3. Why do you want great health and vitality?

4. List five people you consider who live with great health and vitality. How do they live and what can you learn from them?

5. What prevents you from having great health and vitality?

Chapter 2 – Pillar 2: Fulfilling Relationships

Aside from physical health and wellbeing, our relationships have a fundamental impact on our happiness and quality of life. If our relationships are not supporting us, we'll face some tough decisions. Perhaps we might consider a new relationship we would like to create. Shining awareness upon our relationship pillar helps us anticipate the actions necessary to form the relationships we desire. All relationships challenge us at some point. Our task is to constantly analyze our relationships to determine the positive and negative impact they have on our life. From this place we can choose to commit to giving our best self to all relationships we engage in.

The Science of Relationships

According to Dr. Ralph Holloway, a physical anthropologist at Columbia University, the human brain is proportionally larger than other animals due to our complex social interactions. Our brain structure, particularly the temporal lobe region, has evolved to accommodate our many diverse and intricate relationships. Misreading various communication methods, such as body language and tonal inflection, can have unpleasant implications, including arguments, disagreements or physical violence. Our ability to identify and interpret social interactions is expressed in our intimate relationships, friendships, family dynamic, working relationships, or even the seemingly random events of life that draw different people to us. While there are times when we will misread communication signals, developing greater awareness of the unconscious patterns we employ and identifying ways we can address and improve them is part of our development journey.

The personal fulfilment of our relationships is an excellent barometer of the life we are currently living. The quality of the people we regularly and closely engage with goes a long way in determining our levels of success and happiness. If we associate with genuinely successful people with values similar to our own, we will genuinely succeed with our values intact. Period.

Reflecting upon the people closest to us is an activity that can assist in this awareness building process. Just thinking about the people who currently occupy our lives and how much influence they have over our behaviour is powerful. The activity at the end of this chapter asks us to rate these relationships on a scale of 1–10 regarding the happiness and support they currently provide us. It also provides a basis for positive action. We can add more detail to this rating by identifying specific character traits that we choose to associate with or distance ourselves from. Do the people around us have desires for personal improvement and growth similar to ours?

If there are people on our list who rate poorly, it might be time to evaluate the relationship and determine if they are the right people for us. This is tough. Our list of those with lower ratings will most likely include family members, long-term friends and colleagues who we see regularly. If this is the case, while there are some people we can't avoid, we can limit our exposure to them. Our actions might entail an open discussion with them or simply developing a quiet distance. Regardless of our method, taking action to improve the quality of the people who surround us is essential in developing a life on our terms.

Moving around the country and living in different locations has changed the nature of my relationships, as it was easy to remove myself from toxic people and pursue new experiences. It also provided an opportunity to expand the diversity of my relationships. The challenge for all of us is maintaining contact with those people who positively influence our lives once we move away from them.

When moving into new environments, finding the right people can be difficult. At times, I have struck up conversations at train stations, airports and even gone to places where the people I see as positive influences might be, such as sports clubs and investment seminars. Positioning myself where interesting people might be, however, hasn't resulted in much success. People who are fully engaged in their lives are not casually hanging out; they are out there, living great lives. So, in the absence of physically meeting these types of people, I have created a virtual circle of friends.

In my mind, I have created virtual friendships with world class influencers such as Tony Robbins, Les Brown and Gary Vaynerchuk. With little spare time to invest in finding and meeting successful people, looking for positive online influences can be a starting point. By listening to their messages, I am choosing to program my mind to think like them and respond accordingly.

Intimate relationships are the most challenging and rewarding of all relationships we have. We yearn to find someone who can journey through life with us. Finding love is challenging, yet, when we do, we struggle to grow and deepen this connection.

Throughout this book, I will share the seemingly simple actions I take every day to continue to grow an intimate relationship and what I do to take responsibility for making it the very best it can be. We cannot force anything in life and, as much as we may desire a partner, all we can ever really do is place ourselves in a position to allow it to happen.

Mental Models of Relationships

Relationships are complex. We engage with other people and their fluctuating needs and emotional states along with our own. When we were young children at school, it was easier.

If we shared an interest with someone, we were friends; if we shared two things of interest, we were best friends. As we grow older and become socialized, things change. We build mental models of relationships that may not always be based on accurate information and may not always serve our best interests.

Our mental models of relationships are heavily influenced by our experiences as children. The relationships we observed as youngsters are buried so deeply within us, that we might unconsciously replicate those patterns in the present. Our friendships, family and even intimate relationships might still be operating from an outdated narrative that prohibits forward growth in our current relationships. When we grow in our consciousness, we uncover these outdated patterns and find opportunities to take control of our choices within our relationships.

To observe patterns and versions of relationships in our present lives, we can assess the dynamics within our own families. The relationship we have with our family can impact our wellbeing and success on so many levels. Our parents are central to this. During our childhood and young adulthood, our parents create a mental model of who we are and how we should behave. E. M. Pomerantz and R. A. Thompson in their book, Parents' Role in Children's Personality Development, state that up to half of a child's personality is derived from the socialization of parents. They introduced the concept of the psychological resource principle which implies that, combined with our genetic make-up, our parents significantly influence our views and models of the world through their interactions with us and others.

Understanding the scope of this model for ourselves can both assist with our efforts to change as well as present new challenges. Attempting to change or develop ourselves in different ways can create inner conflict with this view of how relationships 'should be'. It can also lead to external conflict as we challenge the relationship models of those we love. Particularly with our parents.

Some parents are blinded by their love for their child that they cannot see them in any different light. Their motivation to keep their child safe in what they perceive as a dangerous world can stagnate or even suffocate the relationship. Some parents are inhibited by their past wounds and perceive their child's desire to grow as a threat. Within these scenarios, it can be difficult for a child to mature with a sense of gratitude for the opportunities and the life itself that has been given to them. Healing and forgiveness can co-exist, however, when adults and their parents reach a place where mutual respect, peace and gratitude converge.

Our parents have provided us with many gifts, and among them is our ability to connect with others as we move out of our home and into the world. In essence, from our parents, we develop a narrative around our relationships and either repeat it or reinvent it as the years pass.

Friendships

Our friendships impact the quality and even the duration of our lives. According to Dan Buettner, Blue Zones founder and National Geographic Fellow, people who have extensive social support groups live longer and healthier than people who don't.

We know we are heavily influenced by our inner circle of friends and as part of our commitment to growth, we need to determine if they are supporting us to become better than we were yesterday and if we are supporting them in the ways they need as well. True relationship is not a one-way street.

Over the last few years, I have become more aware of those in my inner circle. As a result of this reflection, I have made conscious decisions to distance myself from those relationships that aren't life giving. The people that former UK Special Forces (SAS) and author of *Soldier: Respect is Earned* (2020) celebrity Jay Morton would describe as 'drainers'. Those people that drain my energy and enthusiasm. The complainers, the wingers and those so caught up in their mental modelling of life that by simply being in their presence I felt depressed. Instead, I now place my time with the 'radiators'. Those that provide energy, warmth and challenge me to be a better individual.

It takes a significant investment on our part to create and sustain great friendships, particularly as we grow older. Increased demands from children and work commitments decrease the time we can spend with people outside of our families. However, strategies do exist that can help maintain those bonds when time and distance separates.

Specific strategies to maintain and grow this connection with our close friends include sending regular text, voice and video messages of support to them. Purchasing and sending them a book and scheduling time to discuss its contents contributes to their growth as well as ours.

Reflecting on our current friendships to determine which are life-giving and which deter our growth can be engaged regularly. Sometimes our best friends are those who challenge us and expect more from us than we would expect from ourselves. These are the friendships we want to cultivate. So how do we assess them?

A good way to assess the quality of our friendships can be explored through the lens of social penetration theory (SPT) developed by psychologists, Dr. Irwin Altman and Dr. Dalmas Taylor. This concept implies that as relationships develop, so does the level of intimacy that exists between people. The more you get to know people and spend time with them, the deeper the connections and bonds will be. Assessing our friendships through the SPT lens means that our best relationships are those that are continually growing. Determining what that growth looks like is up to each individual. Growth can be found in the friendships that make us laugh, provide permission for us to be ourselves and the ones that challenge us to be a better version of ourselves.

Work Colleagues

Let's consider work colleagues. The people we associate with in our working environment can have a significant impact in shaping our attitudes. Working with positive, uplifting and motivated colleagues can inspire us to deliver more. If our work colleagues are exercising and eating nutritious food, than it can have a positive effect for our habits. The same can occur in poor working environments. If the atmosphere and attitude of employees is poor, there is every chance these habits can affect ours. Fast food lunches and destructive gossip all lead to negative habits that can impact all areas of our lives. The nature of the work we do is neutral. It is our attitude towards the work and the people who surround us that can make any task either a positive life-giving activity or a soul destroying one.

Opportunities for creating great relationships occur all the time. Although we may not always be able to control who comes into our lives, we can learn to manage the relationships closest to us in the most supportive ways. Applying the SPT concept of evaluating our relationships can form the basis for conscious action. From the work we do on ourselves to the effort and authenticity we place on our relationships, it is possible to create fulfilling and supportive connections in the workplace.

Our Rating

Would you choose to be a lover, friend or work colleague with yourself? What rating would you give yourself in these relationship areas? Are you currently bringing your best self to all your closest relationships? The people closet to us, the ones who support us in so many ways may not always be getting the best version of us. We extend care to strangers outside our inner circle daily; the grocer, the service station attendant and the people that randomly cross our path that by the time we arrive home in the evening we are tired and irritable. Our loved ones may not always be getting our best self as much as they should.

Yes, there are times when we will say dumb things and struggle to bring our best to these close relationships, particularly when tired. Yet, our relationship challenge is to remember that the people we love the most, deserve the best relationship care we can provide for them. If we want to have great relationships; intimate, friendships, family and work colleagues we must take the responsibility for creating and sustaining them.

Summary

Relationships require constant work and reflection. No relationship is perfect, and we can always improve them. At their best, our relationships provide joy, love and connection. They are a source of mutual growth and development and have far reaching effects on our happiness. Healthy work relationships enhance productivity, teamwork and collaboration. Supportive friendships allow us to express compassion as well as experience belonging and unity. Through the evolution of our brains, we have developed the capacity to engage with people in complex behaviour patterns. Mastering these patterns, just like a healthy body, require attention and a committed investment.

Activities

1. List the five closest people currently in your life and rate them from 1-10 on how much happiness, joy and support they provide to you.

    1.
    2.
    3.
    4.
    5.

2. Reflect on your intimate relationship and give it a rating of 1-10. What is working and what isn't working in this relationship right now and what ideas do you have to improve it? Are you taking full responsibility in making it the best it can be?

If you are single, reflect on either past relationships or how you feel right now in attracting a life partner. Are you currently in a space where you love yourself so much and feel happy with who you are that you can relax and allow things to happen naturally?

3. What does a great relationship—lover, friend or work colleague look like? What are the characteristics of these relationships that are important for you?

4. Rate yourself as a lover, friend or work colleague and consider the support and encouragement you are providing to those closet to you.

Chapter 3 – Pillar 3: Abundant Finances

Determining our financial success may not seem as important as our health and relationships, and at a foundational level it isn't. Yet, money plays a fundamental role in our lives. Without a good grasp of finances our health and wellbeing will suffer. Many relationships breakdown as a result of financial stress. With financial freedom we can devote the resources required to care for those we love as well as ourselves. Financial success has more to do with our attitude towards wealth and abundance and less do with the actual dollars in our bank account.

Creating Financial Certainty

Mastering the art of accumulating wealth is essential to living life on our terms. Financial independence is the pillar that brings certainty into our lives; certainty in the form of confidence in our ability to meet financial obligations and circulate wealth. We can enjoy our wealth and feel at ease with our financial position.

Without enough money circulating in our lives, we can become fearful of living in scarcity and poverty. Throughout human evolution, our prehistoric brain has developed to scan constantly for potential danger to ensure our survival. In the absence of physical threats, our brain now will focus on potential psychological threats, including a lack of funds in our bank account. Money plays a fundamental role in our lives. If we struggle to pay our monthly bills on time, we'll suffer from stress. Money and financial resources have a have huge impact on the quality of our life.

With financial independence, our ability to support ourselves and others is enhanced. Working through the financial obstacles we have placed along our own path takes dedication and commitment. By obstacle, I mean a learned financial blockage that requires change. These obstacles can be in the form of beliefs that shape our behaviour, misunderstandings regarding our abilities, and unprofitable actions that undermine our goals. This book is a journey in uncovering these obstacles and developing strategies to move beyond these limitations.

Considering obstacles as opportunities establishes a more positive mindset in approaching fear and uncertainty with wealth creation. Too often, we might become distracted and subjected to the language we're using to describe current states that we are experiencing. As a result, we can become limited to the words we use, which then becomes a self-fulfilling prophecy.

The Language of Wealth

The language we use to associate with various states sends powerful messages to ourselves and others about our mindset and our ability to change that state.

Once, I attended a gathering where I overheard a friend say that her father's body had cancer. Her father didn't have cancer; it was his body that had the disease. This example of language, of instilling a powerful separation between a diagnosis and a person assists with our perspective during such challenging times. By distinguishing between her father and the cancer, my friend was able to see beyond her father's physical condition, allowing her to support him as a daughter would want to support her father.

The language of wealth creation can be just as empowering.

Language such as 'I'm broke' or 'I have no money' are labels we tell ourselves about these states, and if we are unaware of this language, we can become trapped by it. Introducing greater awareness of the language we use to describe such states shifts our thinking and builds momentum in making positive changes. The language we use to describe ourselves also reveals beliefs that may not necessarily be serving us.

'Currency' is a term to consider from a fresh perspective in regard to our wealth creation. If we consider what 'current' means, a certain sense of a flow exists, just as it does for water and electricity. Within nature, water flows in a continuous state of directed movement with ease and an electrical impulse is a stream of charged electrons or ions. Currency is also a term used to describe a country's circulation of money and wealth. We can reflect on our relationship to currency. Are we in 'flow' with money? Allowing it to come naturally to us, through us and around us with ease? Or do we resist the natural flow of wealth in and out of our lives and exhaust ourselves trying to keep hold of it?

Many of our beliefs regarding wealth creation come from our observations as youngsters. For many of us, our beliefs impact and may even inhibit our growth as adults. Idioms such as 'money doesn't grow on trees' and 'a penny saved is a penny earned' along with some religious belief systems that associate wealth with greed has translated into a negative mindset around money. These unconscious stories and language associated with money may be sabotaging our actions of creating the financial wealth and abundance we desire.

The term 'frugal' is often associated with wealth creation. This can imply a withholding or a 'Scrooge-like' mentality surrounding wealth creation. Although this belief and pattern of behaviour works for some people, it is time to question this mentality. Frugal comes from the Latin word meaning 'fruit' or 'value' and implies an unwillingness of people to enjoy the fruits of their labour fully. The 'value' part of the word implies some form of virtue associated in this withholding of one's fruits. Interesting, isn't it?

We have taken the word frugal and formed a belief system that there is some virtue in not enjoying our fruits and applied this thinking to the acquisition of wealth. We may come to believe that withholding money and not allowing it to flow around us implies a sense of virtue and unwittingly continue to live with a scarcity mentality throughout our lives. We hold tightly onto what money we receive, fearful of losing it. This mindset inadvertently blocks the natural flow around us. Accepting that there is a universal flow of money and working on our mindset regarding wealth creation can encourage a change of thinking and lead to a change of action.

An example of encouraging the flow of wealth might be investing in a training course that we may have put off due its cost. Perhaps completing the course will present new opportunities through increased knowledge that allows us to increase our cash flow.

By purchasing this book, you are contributing to the flow of wealth in the world and by improving your knowledge, you can magnify your personal wealth. Completing a university degree is another example of the investment we might have to make to increase our salary. The point being, there are many times when sharing our wealth provides opportunities for us to magnify it.

Building Wealthy Beliefs

Challenges around wealth acquisition will almost always exist. From acquiring and circulating more of it in our life to supporting others in their quest for financial independence. Our work is to reach a level of acceptance where we do not judge our 'wealth' by our bank account or material goods, and instead, assess more from our internal beliefs and feelings about it. The work is internal. The work is on ourselves. Our own values, beliefs and mindset around wealth.

Creating habits to develop our awareness around wealth

is the beginning of a deeper inquiry. We can reflect upon our thoughts associated with spending money and the stories we have regarding saving it. This can be exciting work if we choose to make it exciting. Shining a spotlight on how we think, feel and act when we are in positions of spending and receiving money. What is the voice inside you saying when you make financial decisions such as buying a coffee, purchasing a new car or setting money aside for savings? Record these thoughts and feelings in a journal. Ask questions about wealth and how you feel about being wealthy. Imagine yourself as a wealthy person and how you would act, feel and behave.

This is a relationship. Like any relationship, we must take responsibility for growing it in the direction we desire. If we are in a state of unconditional giving in our relationships of love, empathy and compassion, there is a very good chance that this will come back to us at some point. It is the same with our finances. The world is a reverberating place. What we send out to the universe in both a positive and negative way will come back to us in the same form.

Investing our time, energy and resources in understanding more about wealth will improve our appreciation and knowledge of it. Developing an interest in the stock market, housing market or any area that allows wealth to flow into the world grows this relationship. Reading classic books such as *The Instant Millionaire* (1989), *The Richest Man in Babylon* (1926) and *The Millionaire Next Door* (1996) contribute to shaping our mindset towards being wealthy. Seeking guidance from those who have already developed some expertise is another way we can grow our own knowledge.

Taking responsibility for our current situation means we unconditionally accept what has happened in the past and begin to select a new view of wealth creation. We may already possess an abundant amount of 'wealth' yet do not realise or fully appreciate the form that it is in. It could be the knowledge we have acquired over the years or the wisdom we have gained through our unique experiences; appreciating the wealth we already have serves a basis for financial wealth. There are skills that you have acquired throughout your lifetime that many people would benefit from learning. Perhaps now is the time to consider how you can begin to share or capitalize on this wealth.

On the other side of the financial equation, questioning if we genuinely believe that we are worthy of being wealthy can bring up many thoughts and emotions. Consider the type of person you could be if your bank balance was already filled with lots of numbers. How would you treat yourself and those people around you? Continuing to shift our thinking of wealth creation to an internal state of being is a big take away from this book. Understanding that wealth begins with internal development, followed by positive unconditional action leads to great results.

Unconditional action means that we act from a place of wealth and abundance without any expectation of return. It is easy to comprehend, yet difficult to integrate. It's giving the Christmas present without expecting anything back or sharing the knowledge we have with humility and grace. The practice of giving wealth is not a business transaction where we hope to get back what we give (plus extra!). Being truly wealthy on the inside means a state of constant giving without expectation. Giving from this perspective does not only mean money, although that can be a part of it, but also includes our wisdom, our time, our energy, our positivity and our good wishes to all we encounter each day. When was the last time you genuinely complimented a stranger, giving them the very best of yourself without expecting anything in return?

But will all this giving still pay the bills? If we fully believe so yes! Opportunities for wealth creation are unlimited and naturally arise when we are fully aligned with our giving. This occurs only if it truly comes from the heart with selfless intentions.

If our current level of finance is sufficient and already brings a level of comfort and ease, we should begin to look at how we can leverage that mastery into positively impacting the remaining three pillars. Can we begin to invest in a personal trainer to help get our body into better shape? Or can we consult with a stylist to improve our wardrobe? The point being, if one pillar is progressing well, it is logical to leverage that strength into the remaining pillars.

When building momentum to make significant changes in our lives, we first consider the areas that are working for us. I call this the POSITIVE KICK-STARTER APPROACH. It's so much easier to work from this place and leverage from our strengths than working from a disempowered state of observing all our 'failures'. Instead, we focus on what grows for us and use that focus to assist us in other areas of our life.

Modelling Actions of Others

Who is truly wealthy and what characteristics can we model from them? What individual can you think of that you would consider truly wealthy? There is a good chance that the person we think about will not only be financially wealthy but will also live from a place of abundance. Observing people who are genuinely wealthy requires us to see beyond their material wealth. Truly wealthy people live from an internal state of wealth as their money compliments their being. Even if they did not have the big bank balance, they would still be wealthy and most likely acquire money very quickly. Richard Branson is an example of someone who lives from this place of wealth and abundance. A very successful businessman, it's his enthusiasm and energy that truly define his wealth. I'm sure that even if he lost his money tomorrow, he would still have the capacity to amass a great fortune again.

Like the patterns we formed in our relationships at a young age, we have inherited attitudes and emotions regarding wealth. Sometimes those patterns have created limitations in our minds. Now is the time to work with these disempowering beliefs and create new patterns that support us. It's OK to desire financial success and to be clear as to what that entails. It's also important to look at how we can encourage those around us to be just as financially successful, by modeling financial independence ourselves. The concept of being a wealthy person through the mindset we develop and actions we take is central in allowing money to flow to us. Through awareness, deliberate questioning and positive action we can grow our relationship to wealth.

Summary

Financial independence is a worthy goal. The 3rd Pillar of success, creating financial certainty is essential for a fulfilled and happy life. Investigating our beliefs around wealth accumulation are key to making a larger contribution than what we currently contribute. Increasing our awareness around the language we use to describe the status of our wealth experience can allow us to develop this certainty. Accepting there is no virtuosity in living with a scarcity mindset is fundamental in changing our beliefs. Through this internalized work we do on ourselves, we begin to develop the capacity to view wealth acquisition as reflection of our growing consciousness and self-development.

Activities

1. What is your relationship with money and the acquisition of it? Does money come easily to you, or do you find it a constant struggle? What belief or past beliefs do you have that support this story?

2. Review your current finances and gain some clarity around what a 10 looks like for each dimension below.
   - External Reality – Your income, debt, current assets and bank balance.
   - Internal Beliefs – Do you feel wealthy and abundant?
   - Role Models – People you can look to who are currently living a wealth-filled life.

3. Why is an abundance of finances important for you?

4. What prevents you from having abundant finances?

5. Record people who live life from a place of wealth and abundance? Observe their life and research their story for any tips you can apply to yourself.

Chapter 4 – Pillar 4: A Firm Mindset

The dimension of mastering our mindset is the final and possibly most challenging element of the 4 Pillars. Our mindset includes the conscious thoughts we engage each day with along with our unconscious patterns. Our mindset is the invisible maestro pulling the strings of the life we are living and the life that we hope to create. Without a positive and proactive approach to growth, we will never get beyond our current circumstances. With a positive and controlled mindset, we are in control of our thoughts, unshakeable in our actions and centred in our being. We still experience ups and downs in our journey through life, yet we have the capacity to bounce back from setbacks and continue towards our dreams and desires.

Speaker, pastor and author, Eric D. Thomas wrote: 'If there is no enemy within, the enemy outside can do us no harm.' Imagine that for a moment—no enemy within. No self-doubt, no fear, no anxiety and no little voice that is constantly telling us what we can and can't do.

Friend or Foe?

Is your mind your enemy or your friend? If you are like many people, the answer might be the enemy; particularly in the areas where we face our biggest challenges. Our mind can be set against us in achieving the health, wealth, and abundance we desire, and it uses every trick it can to identify why we can't improve a situation. If there is something on the news about economic tightening, it will whisper to us; if there is a bill that comes in the mail, it will speak to us; and when we check our bank balance, it will scream that we can't achieve our desires. These same conversations are incessant in all the pillars. Conscious or not, these negative conversations are repeatedly played within our mind resulting in unproductive habits and results.

We need to take back control of our thoughts.

Consider our mind a garden that requires constant work and attention to keep it looking at its best. The weeds—or negative thoughts—naturally spring up and overrun our garden if we allow them. Like any good gardener, time and energy needs to be invested in pulling those negative weeds. Also, as any good gardener knows, we must be careful of which seeds we plant. These seeds (or thoughts) require a lot more effort to remove once established. Sometimes, it is winter in our garden, and it appears that nothing beautiful will ever grow again. Sometimes, we feel that our garden is in a total state of bloom and will forever be that way. Life in the garden teaches us however, that everything has a season, and we must attend to it daily.

To get our minds working with us and not against us is strategized in this book. From positive self-talk and journaling to taking small risks every day, we can condition our psyche to believe that we are capable of more. From introducing new habits and rituals into our lives, to seeking assistance from the people around us, there are many ways we can begin to take back control of our destiny.

Like everything in life, it is important to experiment. Find the fun in the challenges and if it works, stick with it. If it doesn't, discard. Over time, you can take on bigger challenges.

Mental Illness

Mental illnesses such as depression, anxiety and trauma-related disorders are affecting more people. According to Ohio State University journalist, Rubina Kapil and her article on the Mental Health First Aid website in 2019, almost half of American adults (46.4%) will experience a mental illness during their lifetime. How is it that in developed countries such as Australia, USA and Britain, mental illness and suicide rates are so high, particularly among the young? Something is wrong within society that is harming our mental health.

As our brains have evolved to look for danger and our prehistoric minds have been conditioned to look for fear, over time, this pattern can deepen to the detriment of our mental health. We evolved from hunters and gatherers trying to avoid being eaten, and we are still unconsciously scanning our environment for danger. Depending on the challenges we face, these 'dangers' may be directed towards ourselves when looking in the mirror and criticizing what we see. We can assume our friends or colleagues are talking about us behind our back or experience a spike of anxiety when an unexpected bill arrives. The threats created in our mind can appear as our reality. It is our mind that has made these experiences so threatening.

To free ourselves from negative thinking and take positive action, we must constantly work on our mindset. This takes time and consistent effort. Changing our mindset and overcoming a particular thought pattern can take months or years. At the same time, it's also possible to change our mindset in a moment. Perhaps from time invested in clearing away negative and unproductive thoughts or the result of a significant life event. People can change with the right leverage. For some that is a health challenge, for others, family can be the primary motivator for change.

Learning to relax and release thoughts as the occur is another process to free ourselves from negative thinking. Michael Singer, in his *New York Times* bestseller *The Untethered Soul* (2007), describes a state of being where through attention and consistent practice we can breathe and relax unproductive thoughts before they become fixed in our mindset. It's taking a step back from an event and allowing it to pass before getting caught in it. A car beeps at us while driving and we take a moment to let it pass without going into a mental conversation that lasts with us for the rest of the day. This state of centred being occurs once we make the decision to detach from our thoughts and observe the interactions within our mind with care and awareness.

RAS

What is your mindset right now? Is there a dominant thought pattern or feeling that is consistently arising for you and impacting your body, your relationships or finances? Are you living with past thoughts or in future predications? Neuroscientist Rick Hanson provides the analogy in *Buddha's Brain* (2009) that negative experiences stick in our brains like Velcro, while positive experiences, such as receiving a compliment from a stranger, slide off like Teflon. This supports that what we repeatedly think, with most of it being negative, tends to become ingrained into our being. The Reticular Activation System (RAS) is a series of filters located within the brain that sifts information and discards what is irrelevant or unimportant. If we choose to constantly focus on all the positive events that are occurring in our life our brain will automatically respond by looking for the positive.

The key here is focus. We can easily distract ourselves with media, particularly social media, and the bombarding messages that call for our attention. The constant messages that we must attain the perfect body, model spouse, and million-dollar home are all avenues for comparison and judgement. It takes a concerted effort to remove these distractions and take control of the information flooding our minds. Fortunately, with a little awareness, we can recognize these distractions and direct our mind towards the destinations we choose.

The RAS is the same system that draws our attention to the make of car we are looking to purchase when buying. As our thoughts are focused on a particular make/model, our brain will automatically draw these cars to our attention when driving. All of a sudden, it seems as though every car we pass is the exact same model of the one we are looking to purchase.

However, we must do the work to train our mind to focus on productive concepts rather than negative patterns of thinking. Ingrained negative patterns make working with our mindset the most challenging of the 4 Pillars. Often it is difficult to see the external results that we are putting into our mindset, and it can quickly fluctuate between positive and negative states. We cannot hide from our mind, as it knows all our tricks and can turn our best intentions into self-deprecating, ego-driven sabotage. If properly trained, it can also inspire our thoughts and actions to overcome any obstacle as the most powerful ally we can ever have.

In many ways, we can feel both trapped and freed by this powerful ally. It takes great courage to open the Pandora's box and explore our mind. Our thoughts are often messy and illogical. Yet our mindset holds the key to unlocking our potential. Interestingly, the goal or purpose of yoga, as described by the great sage Patanjali, is *Chitta vritti nirodhah*, which when translated from Sanskrit literally means, 'Yoga is the removal of the fluctuations of the mind.' The desired union that comes from the cessation of this fluctuating mind talk is the goal of oneness and unity that we can apply in all areas of life.

Awareness

Developing awareness of the internal dialogue is the first step. Our goal is to control and focus our mindset towards the areas that are important for us while removing distractions. This is the two-step journey: remove distractions while channeling our efforts towards our goals.

This is not an easy task and requires fine tuning of our attention. Scheduling time to watch, listen and learn more about our mindset is the only path towards gaining control over it. Growing an awareness of our thoughts allows us to develop an understanding and question what is really going on inside. Through building our awareness, we can link our actions to our thoughts and see the impact they are having on us. For example, when you woke up this morning, can you remember some of the first thoughts that entered your mind? Were they positive about the day ahead or were they negative about an impending problem that you had to solve? Often those first few thoughts in the morning carry over from our last thoughts the previous evening. If we can begin to steer these thoughts in a more positive direction, we are beginning to set ourselves up for a more positive mindset. It is simple to comprehend yet takes dedication and courage to train the mind in this way. The smallest of changes in focus, when habitual and consistent, have the most powerful implications on our lives.

Where we begin our observations of the first few moments of waking in the morning, we might notice that our mind immediately focuses on the difficulties facing us that day. It could range from having to get out of a warm and comfortable bed, to traffic congestion, or a million other worries or 'problems' that we face.

After continual practice, patience and with awareness, we can choose to focus on these things—or something else. We can become the gardener of our mind. Although negative thoughts (weeds) still come to our attention, we are in control of how we react to them. Do we give in to them and let them determine our state? Or do we choose to focus on something more positive? Most of the time, the reality behind the thoughts that enter our minds is never quite as bad as our mind makes it out to be. So why give them time?

What we give our attention usually has a way of unfolding for us and it's easier to be aware of these thoughts first thing in the morning when all around us is still quiet. Consider rising early in the morning, when distractions in our mind are few. When we aim to develop an awareness of our thoughts and where we place our attention, we develop a foundation for changing our actions for the better. If we are not conscious of the internal dialogue, then we can have less control over evolving towards a healthier, richer direction.

As an example, when we have a particularly challenging conversation coming up with a colleague, our mind will naturally focus on the impending discomfort of that conversation, making it difficult to focus on other things. Our thoughts anticipate this future conversation, clouding our judgment and even our ability to think positively about it. We also know that after these conversations, our mind will continually replay the event with alternative scenarios and responses that may or may not have been more effective.

Instead of allowing our mind to grind away with worry and the anticipation of negative outcomes, strive to control the negative thoughts before and after the conversation through action. Before the conversation, write out bullet points of what you need to say and how you anticipate your colleague to respond. Even role play with a trusted friend. If you feel nervous, go for a run or listen to music. Once fully prepared, let go of the situation and just wait for it. And then, once the conversation is completed, know you have done your best. Consciously choosing where we place our focus is the goal. Maintaining that focus, like a muscle we train in the gym, requires practice, repetitions and the ability to draw this focus back into our control.

Developing strategies we can implement to develop our focus, control our mindset, and shift negative thoughts to positive ones are beneficial. Activities such as intense physical activity, expressing gratitude to others, concentration training (or meditation) and breath work can assist in getting our mind back into a positive and peaceful state. Recording our thoughts through journal writing can provide an opportunity to strengthen our awareness building capacity along with providing a creative outlet for these thoughts.

Our mindset is the highest bastion of self-development work. The work is not easy. It is continuous. There is no other greater pathway to master than through mastery of one's mindset. Our mind will fluctuate between thoughts quickly, sometimes within microseconds. However, if we are serious about improving ourselves and mastering the 4 Pillars, then we must develop an appreciation and awareness of what is happening inside our mind. We will become objective enough to watch these thoughts and consciously choose where we place our focus, implementing strategies to redirect our mind when it is distracted. Our mindset can be our greatest ally if we begin the process of training it to be.

Summary

Working with our mindset is the most challenging of the 4 Pillars. Our minds and corresponding senses have wandered freely to focus on whatever is most appealing at any one time. This constant external distraction is impacting the life we desire and our sense of happiness and joy. Working on our mindset is a long-term project. With a controlled, positive mindset, however, the remaining 3 Pillars are easier to master, and we can direct ourselves towards the future we desire.

Activities

1. Reflect on your mindset and describe below what a rating of 10 would look like for each of the following dimensions.

- Current mindset – can you conduct a positive/negative ratio?
- Awareness of your thoughts – first thing in the morning
- Awareness of your thoughts – on a daily basis
- How quickly your mind can let go of negative events?
- How much time do you devote to working on your mindset?

2. What are the 5 major sources of distraction in your life?

3. How much of your thinking is concerned with future thoughts are past experiences?

4. How important (on a scale of 1-10) is it for you to have a firm and controlled mindset?

5. What currently prevents you from having a controlled mindset?

Chapter 5 – Ritualize to Actualize

How we spend our time determines the quality of our lives. From the moment we rise in the morning until we fall asleep at night, we are forming our future based on our actions throughout the day. There are 86,400 seconds in each day. How we choose to spend those seconds shapes who we become and the life we lead.

We Become What We Repeatedly Do

At this moment in time, you are the direct result of the actions you have previously taken. From the state of your health to your relationships and mindset, your past actions are being seen today. You may have consciously chosen to act on your health in the past through exercising on a regular basis or you may have unconsciously chosen inaction. Inaction can be more detrimental than taking inappropriate action. Not acting equals ignorance. We can no longer use ignorance as an excuse when creating a life on our terms.

Creating a life on our terms and achieving mastery of the 4 Pillars requires us to become extraordinary people. To become extraordinary people, we must live in an extraordinary state. To live in an extraordinary state, we must have extraordinary habits and rituals. Our habits and rituals form the foundation for the life we are creating. Therefore, we need to analyse our time and determine if our activities support us in the direction we would like to go. From this process, we can introduce new habits or modify our existing habits to realize more of our potential.

It can be challenging to let go of an existing habit or behaviour pattern, particularly when old habits are so ingrained and easily repeated. Society and culture may also be reinforcing these not so positive habits—messages that say it's OK to have those chocolate biscuits to pep us up in the afternoon, or that we deserve to sleep in a little longer because we had a late night. Messages like these are so deeply embedded within us, that it takes conscious effort to analyze our behaviours and create new ones. Our mind is also an expert at seeking 'quick-fix' messages. It is conditioned to seek comfort and use whatever tactic it can to lull us onto the easy path. Deep satisfaction, though, arises from creating new rituals that lead to new results.

At this point, a distinction between habits and rituals can help support our goals. A habit, by definition, is any activity performed routinely without conscious effort or thought. We all have our daily habits such as brushing our teeth, combing our hair or going to sleep on a particular side of the bed each night. None of these habits can be classified as either 'good' nor 'bad'; they are patterns of behaviour that we follow without much thought.

Then there are habits that can be considered positive or negative depending on the impact they have on our lives. Choosing to eat healthy or unhealthy on a regular basis is one example of a habit we have formed over time that generally doesn't take much effort on our part to continue. Depending on what we put on our plate for each meal and the quality of its nutrients, we could classify our dietary intake as having either a positive or negative impact on our health.

The same principle of habits applies to our fitness regime, relationships, finances and mindset. Over time, we create unconscious patterns of behaviour that have become so normal that we don't even realize we are doing them. Unconscious habits such as having the last word in an argument or impulse buying when a sale is on. It doesn't matter what the habit is, developing awareness around that habit and determining if it serves us is the path of progress.

Rituals

Rituals can be considered activities that are performed with awareness or for the purpose of developing awareness. Often associated with religious devotion, rituals are activities we choose to do to bring us closer to being the person we want to be. A ritual might be taking a few moments before falling asleep at night in gratitude. It would be considered a ritual because it requires us to bring conscious thought into our awareness for the purpose of reflection and gratitude.

Further rituals we could create involve how we speak with our partner when things become tense or taking a walk when a sale pops up on our screen. These types of rituals are 'circuit breaker' rituals. They provide an opportunity for awareness in a space that would otherwise entail unconscious reactions. Sometimes we need to enlist the support of others when creating new rituals, as it is very easy to fall back into old patterns, particularly when under pressure or things don't go our way.

Even though rituals are commonly associated with religious groups, many individuals, companies and successful sporting teams use rituals to connect meaning with daily activities. One of the most successful sporting teams throughout history, the New Zealand All Blacks use rituals to connect new players to the group, the group to the country and the country to its culture. The traditional Maori Haka performed before a test match is the ultimate ritual in preparing the team and country for battle. James Kerr, in *Legacy* (2013), describes many of the symbolic rituals the All Blacks implement to maintain their status as the best in the world. Kerr uses the term, 'Ritualize to Actualize' as a powerful reminder that the rituals we perform on a daily basis help us in 'actualizing' our goals.

Awareness and intention are the clear distinctions between a habit, an unconscious set of behaviours, and a ritual. Developing awareness of our habits is the first step in discriminating between habits that support us and habits that require change. Creating rituals to support the change we want to make is fundamental when learning to master the 4 Pillars. Experimenting with those rituals is a good way to determine if they are effective for us.

Enjoy experimenting with new rituals. These can be learnt from podcasts, books, or highly accomplished individuals. Constant reflection on your own habits and making small changes to your routines to support your goals keeps things fresh and new. This is not always a simple process. There will be times when you fall back into past habits and must modify new rituals to sustain them. Habits involving nutrition can be particularly challenging as food satisfies many of our emotional needs as well. Sometimes it will feel that we take two steps forward only to regress a step or two, impacting our motivation and mindset. Accepting these setbacks as part of the journey and refocusing on our desires can make the transition to new rituals easier.

Fortunately, when creating new rituals, there is a good chance they will eventually become habits if we commit to performing them with full consciousness. The length of time in the journey from ritual to unconscious habit will vary depending on how big a change we are making but consistency is essential. For example, if we decide we would like to go to sleep a little earlier or rise a little earlier in the morning, we will need a clear reason why we would like to create this new ritual and be consistent in performing it.

There should also be some new rituals we create that should never be turned into a habit. We don't want our morning meditation to become a habit for us, where we feel we must get it done to feel complete for the day. That defeats the entire intention behind a ritual. If we reflect that a ritual is a practice performed with religious devotion, we must distinguish between those new routines we would like to become a habit, and those that form part of our morning rituals.

A ritual that I have turned into a habit is taking a cold shower each morning. I do this as a reminder to myself and my mind that I am in control of my decisions and that I have the power to control my actions. The physiological and psychological benefits of cold showers are many. Wim Hof, also known as 'The Iceman', has been the subject of many scientific studies examining the impact of cold-water immersion on the body and mind. Radboud University Medical Centre and the Academic Medical Centre Amsterdam of The Netherlands and Wayne State University School of Medicine are among the groups who have studied Wim Hof's claims. These studies confirm that cold water immersion improves the body's physical immune response by increasing the amount of white blood cells, enhance alertness through oxygen saturation of cells and reduces stress. Psychological benefits include increased willpower. Weight loss has also been associated with cold water immersion through increased metabolic rate. This ritual may not be for everyone, however, by consciously choosing to get into a cold shower, I have already won a small battle with my mind. Taking a cold shower is not what I want to do at 4 a.m. in winter. At that hour, my mind is having an internal conversation about how stupid this is. I might get a cold, the flu or that no 'normal' person would be awake doing this. This internal conversation is always present. And each day, I jump into the shower, turn on the cold tap and try to enjoy the experience for a few minutes.

And you know what? I always feel good for doing it no matter how cold I feel during or afterwards. I think this has more to do with the fact that I have won that first battle with my mindset for the day. Through this activity, I feel that I am in control of my day, and I am advancing towards my goals. This ritual has become so ingrained in my daily routine, that it is now easier to have a cold shower than a warm one. Yes, the internal voice still tries to dissuade me, but its volume has gotten quieter over time.

Through sharing these habits and rituals, my aim is to provide ideas for you to find inspiration in creating your own daily rituals. We often learn from the example of others. There is no specific rule book to follow when creating and experimenting with rituals, however each of us must begin where we are and with what we have. It can be easy to use our current job or situation as an excuse for not creating positive habits but truly, the 'perfect' time is now.

Creating new rituals is challenging and the path of progress is never linear. We go through stages when we get on a roll and make great progress with our body, relationship, finances, and our mindset. We also endure setbacks and challenges. Yet, remaining the same and repeating the same mistakes can be more disheartening than the fear of change.

Some of these habits and rituals may not be for everyone. Use your own judgement and experiment with different rituals to explore this challenge. There could be some new rituals you could implement today, and you will notice an immediate positive impact in your life. While there will be other rituals that will never reflect the person you are or the person you are becoming.

Be on the lookout for new rituals and have the courage to try new things. This attitude toward growth is central in mastering the 4 Pillars. Creating rituals is an exciting process with the right attitude. Consider it an opportunity for you to add more into your life with the activities that benefit you. You are consciously creating a new you from these activities and it is empowering.

My rituals and habits shared below have evolved over time.

I am continuously on the lookout for new rituals as some work for a period until they are replaced, while others have been a foundational part of my day for years.

Creating Morning Rituals

As I shared in the opening pages of this book, early morning is my time to plan for success. What I do in those first hours has a lasting impact on my performance for the rest of the day. It may appear contradictory that certain activities early in the morning provide stamina to last the entire day, yet these activities energize my body and calm my mind.

Our rituals do not have to be amazing feats of physical exertion or take hours to complete. What is important is the intention behind them and their consistency. Setting aside 30 minutes of 'me' time may be a challenge early on. Start small— even with ten minutes—and achieve success there first with a realistic goal, before setting aside hours and feeling guilty for not completing all your activities. Small, consistent steps over long periods result in amazing achievements and the mindset we aim to cultivate.

My first ritual after my alarm sounds is to focus my mind on something positive. It can be something I am anticipating that day or a general gratitude for something specific. I often focus on one area of the 4 Pillars such as a moment of gratitude for my health, my relationship or something as simple as how fortunate I am to have a bed to sleep in.

Once out of bed, I drink something alkaline such as wheatgrass, barley grass or spirulina to hydrate the body and alkalize it after several hours of fasting. According to a study conducted by Mujoriya & Bodla in *Food Science and Quality Management* (2011), wheatgrass has been attributed to many health benefits including increasing immunological activity, reducing oxidative stress and even potentially eliminating cancer cells. Drinking filtered water first thing in the morning can help hydrate every cell in our body and give it the best start possible to reach its optimal state. Being dehydrated affects our body and its energy levels throughout the day and impacts our cognitive and problem-solving abilities. The Zazen Alkaline water system, or a similar device, is my recommended water system. It filters toxins and bacteria from tap water and alkalizes and energizes the water with minerals found in nature.

A recent ritual that has become an integral addition to my morning routine is having a coffee with my partner. The organic fair-trade beans are blended with MCT/coconut oil, reishi powder and ghee. 'Bulletproof Coffee' is a combination of fats from the coconut oil and ghee, together with the stimulating effects of coffee. Although conflicting evidence exists on the benefits of drinking this combination, studies have concluded that benefits may include increased mitochondrial and brain function. Adding a small teaspoon of high-quality Chaga powder, a medicinal mushroom that supports health and vitality, I set my body up for the day ahead and spend a little time with my partner.

Over our coffee, my partner and I have an opportunity to read together, discuss our reflections and share our thoughts. Sometimes we share what we have read and discuss the implications in our lives. Other times we will discuss the upcoming day or what is currently occupying our minds. These conversations provide a space for deeper connections and allow us to be present with each other before commencing our day.

After coffee, I move on to the computer for 20 minutes of writing. Twenty minutes is not much time from an entire day to devote to something that cultivates the person I want to become. While I may not always produce a huge volume of work, this time is important in developing a new mindset in the cycle of continual improvement. This is my time to work on projects that are of interest to me.

After 20 minutes of writing, it's onto 10-15 minutes of breath work that I have developed to open the lungs, warm up the body and clear out my nasal passages. It's a combination of ancient yogic breathing techniques along with breath retention. Our breath is so fundamental to our health yet so easily overlooked by most people. Try exhaling and see how long you can hold your breath and we begin to realize how important it is. The average person takes around 20,000 breaths per day so just imagine what a little more oxygen could do to our cells, metabolism and mindset?

Also, as many illnesses are viral, maintaining fully functioning and clean lungs helps fight off diseases such as the common cold and flu. The Wim Hof Method is a great place to start in learning the foundations of breath work.

Once the breath work is completed it's into the cold shower and then the yoga mat for 60 minutes of Ashtanga Yoga. This challenging practice has taken a long time to learn, however I have noticed a considerable improvement in many areas of my life as a result of this comprehensive system. It's not the easiest form of yoga, but I feel so wonderful afterwards that it's worth the daily effort. I usually complete this practice 4–6 times per week, depending on how I feel, but I always ensure that I have at least one day of complete rest throughout the week.

Like everything we do, balance is important, and exercise should be the same. The variety of strength building through lifting weights and flexibility training with Ashtanga Yoga means that I can maintain muscle strength while increasing range of motion. Alternating between high-intensity interval training (HIIT) and long slow jogs/rowing machine activity to maintain cardiovascular fitness is important but never underestimate the benefits of walking for both our body and mind.

The physical exercise we do, and the variety of those movements should change as we change. Ageing bodies require a greater level of care and sensitivity. Competing with younger individuals in any physical activity is an ego driven exercise and a recipe for injury. We can, however, continually challenge ourselves to improve our fitness as we age. Our physical body responds to the demands we place upon it. If we fail to move our body in appropriate ways, it will deteriorate to the extent that we become limited in our capacity to enjoy life. Incorporating a variety of movement, intensity and duration as we age assists the body to maintain vitality to meet our changing energetic demands.

The final part of my morning ritual is to sit in meditation for some quiet time. The length of time varies, yet this time withdraws my consciousness from the external world, allowing me to recover from physical activity and concentrate my mind. Benefits of meditation are numerous, particularly in times of stress. Scientists from the *Irish Journal of Psychological Medicine* have found that mindfulness-based stress reduction (MBSR) techniques have shown meditation to reduce anxiety, depression and pain-scores. There are many apps available (e.g., Insight Timer) for guided meditations for stress relief and relaxation as well as mindfulness techniques for improving awareness and focus. Remember, it's not about how 'perfect' we are or how deep we go, it's about including meditation into our morning rituals.

With these habits and rituals, I set myself up to be in the most energizing state possible for the day ahead. I devoted time to progressing my body, my relationship and my mindset and have set the foundation for an extraordinary life. Through devoting time on each of these pillars early in the morning, I can leave my house assured that regardless of what happens for the rest of the day, I am still moving forward in the areas that are important for me.

Key Rituals

- Focus on something positive
- Drink filtered water and alkalizing greens
- Spend quality time with your partner
- Devote 20 minutes to a passion project
- Exercise the body
- Meditate

Summary

Creating a life on our terms requires us to live an extraordinary life. Exploring new rituals and habits to support this progresses us closer in mastering the 4 Pillars and creating a life on our terms. No one ritual or habit is more important than another but in combination, these activities determine the life we create. Be open to experimenting with rituals and learn from others to provide guidance and inspiration. Our goal is to prioritize the rituals we create and develop consistency in making continual progress.

Activities

1. Construct two columns on a page with the headings, 'Supportive Habits' and 'Unsupportive Habits.' List 10–15 of your daily habits that fall under these categories. Begin from the moment you wake up until you fall asleep each night.

2. What are some new rituals you can begin to create in each of the 4 Pillars? For each of the pillars below, list 2-3 new rituals you can implement immediately to support you in the direction you want to go.

- Body
- Relationship
- Finances
- Mindset

3. What is it important for you to implement these new rituals?

4. What would prevent you from implementing these new rituals?

5. List some 'circuit breaker' activities you can perform in each of the 4 Pillars that you can use to enhance your awareness when faced with challenges.

Chapter 6 – Small Changes Equal Big Results

To prevent feeling overwhelmed with the process of change, examining various change processes and applying the one that best aligns with your desires is your best strategy. When we think about change from different perspectives, we develop control over this process. If we feel we are in control of the changes we are implementing, then we are more likely to succeed.

The 1% Rule

The 1% Rule or the 'marginal gains approach' was inspired by former English track cycling coach Sir David Brailsford. His philosophy of focusing on the tiny, almost insignificant elements that go into riding a bicycle, resulted in the English team claiming seven out of 10 gold medals on the track in both the 2008 Beijing and 2012 London Olympics. From improving bike mechanics, the aerodynamics of helmets, biomechanics of riders and even traveling with team pillows, every element of an athlete and team performance was broken down into small, manageable components. From those small components, 1% improvement was sought.

The 1% Rule is supported by what we know about the workings of the brain. If the change we undertake is significant, it has the potential to threaten the brain's comfortable and predictable pattern. The amygdala can fire, and the 'flight, fight or freeze' part of the brain reacts. We can use will power and motivation to override this primitive defense mechanism for only so long and may eventually succumb to failure. Through the 1% Rule, we can choose to accomplish small habits and rituals so that the brain is not threatened, increasing our chances of success.

Consider how ten 1% changes would be an overall improvement of 10% is worth remembering when introducing new rituals. The key is choosing one small element from each of the 4 Pillars and implement a change routine that will only take a little effort on your part. This gradual shift may be difficult to start, particularly if we have suffered previous setbacks, but if we easily achieve several small victories, we improve our mindset and will naturally seek larger challenges.

A small 1% ritual that you may implement for continual improvement in your relationship is to leave a note for your partner each day before you leave for work. This note will take less than 1 minute to write but sends a message that you love him and look forward to being home again with him. He will read the note before you arrive home and it will help with his mindset regardless of the day he has had. A 1% effort can make a significant impact on a relationship.

New Year's resolutions rarely last longer than a week or two as drastic changes are too overwhelming. Instead, we work with the mind when introducing change and use our knowledge to foster success. Initially we take on small tasks to build the foundation of success and inspiration that leads to larger challenges. Positive self-talk strategies, or repeatedly telling ourselves that an activity is temporary or trying something new is fun, trains the mind and gives us control over our focus.

If the change we are making is minor, this internal positive self-talk works long enough to establish a routine and to identify positive outcomes consciously. For example, we may feel healthier from drinking filtered water or our sleep may improve from purchasing that new pillow. When our mind associates the change with a positive outcome, we are on a winner.

Little things really do make a difference and the concept of the Compound Effect, written by Darren Hardy, illustrates how to make successful changes. It is very easy to think that small changes won't impact our overall picture of great health and vitality, but it is attention to detail that sets society's leaders like Elon Musk and Bill Gates apart.

The Compound Effect states that little actions performed over a long period of time have a significant impact on the end result. That chocolate bar every afternoon at work equates to approximately 2,600 bars over 10 years or 30 kg of extra body fat. That one chocolate bar each day can have such an astonishing result!

Consider applying the Compound Effect to your health, your relationships and your finances. Little gestures each day to remind your partner how much you love them or save a few extra dollars each week. In financial terms, compound interest is the 'secret' that has seen Warren Buffett accumulate 99% of his fortune after the age of 50. Even Albert Einstein called it 'the eighth wonder of the world.' We all want the big, glamorous story and forget that to create a big outcome, little tasks were consistently performed.

Neglecting the 1% Rule can also have a significant impact on our life over time. Our relationship is an example of how we can begin to neglect these seemingly little things that can lead to long-term disaster. Most people at the beginning of an intimate relationship find great joy in doing little things such as sending messages, having dinners out or just being present with their partner. However, over time, as they begin to take these relationships for granted, they can neglect the 1% activities until the relationship deteriorates and no longer works.

Our success or failure in mastering the 4 Pillars is determined by these 1% activities. These little things accumulate an enormous impact over time. The quality of people in our inner circle also has a significant impact on us devoting the time necessary to change for the better. If our friends are neglecting their ability to change and grow, so will we.

By paying attention to the 1% details, we are distinguishing ourselves from others. Furthering a mindset that will naturally lead to greater opportunities. Opportunities that don't come to those who are unprepared for them.

Establishing a New Habit

How long does it take for a change of behaviour or new ritual to become part of our routine? That depends on some factors. According to Scott Frothingham in healthline.com, anywhere between 18 days up to 254 days for people to establish a consistent shift. There is also the popular 21/90 rule that states that a habit is formed over a period of 21 consecutive days and then reinforced over the next 90 days.

Our mindset and the story we tell ourselves towards any change is central to creating a life on our terms. Society is littered with examples of people who lost an amazing amount of weight only to regain it or lottery winners who quickly lost their winnings. Unless we are prepared to do the inner work, the outer reality we experience quickly reverts back to what it originally was. Sure, our external view of the world can change through such events, but lasting change is staked in the deep, internal shifts of our mindset or beliefs.

Do we really want to improve our body, our relationship or our finances? Do we begin to see progress, but something always happens and before we know it, we have slipped back into old patterns? The external event that triggered the relapse is not important; the fact that setbacks keep occurring is and needs our exploration.

Unless there is alignment between our goals and our internal beliefs, trying to change is like trying to hold a balloon underwater. We can use all our willpower to keep it under the water, but eventually we will run out of that calibre of force and the moment that happens, the balloon automatically springs back to the surface. The larger the balloon (or change), the more willpower required to keep the balloon underwater. Therefore, why make the process of change so hard by undertaking too many changes at once?

The Kaizen Approach

Kaizen is a Japanese word that means continual improvement or refinement and has been used as a basis for company improvement since the 1980s. Toyota car manufacturing company is probably the best-known example of the principle in action, and it is a natural fit when considering the process of change.

The theory works on the basis that change within an organization is an ongoing process. There is always room for improvement and every person has a responsibility to be a part of that improvement. Now, considering when this theory first gained popularity, the idea that every person was responsible for change and refinement was revolutionary. Traditionally, change rested in the hands of the managers and supervisors and the role of the factory worker was to carry out their task without question.

The Kaizen approach assumes that each person is responsible for change. That response can be positive, negative or no response at all (negative response). Positive progress comes from positive responses. How can we continually look for ways to 'refine' our positive habits? First, there are no quick fixes. A tendency to look for the fast, easy options erode resilience and grit. True, lasting and consistent change requires an application of Kaizen approach.

Successful UCLA Basketball coach John Wooden was an example of the Kaizen approach in action. His belief in applying oneself in becoming a little better each and every day over a period of time resulted in an unprecedented 10 NCAA championships. What many don't realize is that it took 16 years of continual improvement before Wooden won his first National Championship.

If we fully apply the Kaizen approach to our lives, we realize the journey never ends. We are never finished with our work. The 'I'll be happy when...' syndrome is symptomatic of a person and society who believes that all their problems will be solved when an external change occurs in their circumstance. However, even in the unlikely scenario that an external change does happen, unless our internal mindset shifts, we'll almost always float back to that state where our minds and beliefs are most comfortable.

Does this mean we shouldn't try to initiate change, as it is so challenging? Should we adhere to the Bart Simpson approach of 'can't win, don't try'?

If a masterpiece of art takes many years to complete, what shifts inside us when we see our lives as a masterpiece in progress? As the saying goes, 'The harder the battle, the sweeter the victory.' For those of us out there battling away on self-development, the feeling of victory when we do accomplish a goal or instil change after many months of effort is true fulfilment. The sweet little victories will bring us the most joy and happiness.

Failing to Success

How many times should we fail in changing or creating a new habit or ritual before we give up? For most people, it takes 3-4 failures before they resign themselves to the fact that they cannot change a habit. The concept of failing towards success is a poignant reminder that every great achiever overcame setbacks on their journey.

History is littered with examples of people who faced great adversity and challenges to become who they were. Former Presidents (Abraham Lincoln), athletes (Michael Jordan), scientists (Albert Einstein) and television personalities (Oprah Winfrey) have all overcome many obstacles and failures in their path to achieving greatness.

We will encounter many setbacks in the process of changing a habit or creating a new ritual—this is a part of the process. Once we resign ourselves to this reality, it's easier to continue to progress. If our setbacks are seen as an integral part of the learning process, the real test comes in our response to our setbacks. Do we try again? Perhaps change our approach?

The meaning we associate with setback is more important than the setback itself. If we classify a setback as a catastrophe, then we respond accordingly, triggering the amygdala. However, if we associate setback with learning and growth, we have an opportunity to respond positively. The language we associate with the event impacts how our brain and consequently our emotions will react.

A financial challenge is an example that can easily be perceived as a detrimental setback. If we have lost money through an investment decision or debt, there are two ways we can respond. We can feel fear with every purchase and belittle ourselves with negative self-talk. Or we can take control of our mindset, look to the lessons that we learned and take positive action, both in our mindset and through our actions.

Yes, it is easy to write these words, but we can always find positive meaning from the events in our lives if we look hard enough. It is tough work. Particularly when we endure challenges over a long period of time. However, just like the examples of the successful people above, as long as we can still breathe, there is time and opportunity for us to succeed.

Setbacks affect our pride, our ego and fuel our negative mindset. It is normal to fear failure, but that fear can prevent us from taking the risks necessary for change. It takes courage to create new rituals and habits and that courage is tested when we are confronted with setbacks. If we condition ourselves to associate a more positive meaning with setbacks, primarily through the language we associate with it, then we are crafting a foundation for our new action, and for a life we choose to create.

Our WHY Matters

Developing a clear understanding of our 'why' also assists in our journey. Our purpose lies at the very centre of almost all the actions we take. We are motivated to take action to improve our lives, so it is wise to review these reasons consciously.

Why do you want to make changes to your rituals and habits in the first place? Are the reasons strong enough to keep you moving forward no matter what? Understanding our primary reasons for our actions keeps us strong in times of challenge. If our desire to reduce our weight is to fit into our summer clothes, we will probably struggle to succeed. Our 'why' is simply not compelling enough. However, if our doctor informed us that we need to get in shape now or we won't be around to see our child's wedding, we will be determined to make the changes.

The words 'motivation' and 'drive' are often used regarding change yet rarely understood. Motivation comes from the Latin word *movere* or motive, indicating a reason to move. We can be motivated to do or move anything on a short-term basis, such as going for a walk or eating a healthy snack. However, when we are driven, we are called in a much deeper way. Drive is a calling for action. Drive can literally move mountains. When we are driven to accomplish something, such as changing a habit or creating a new ritual, nothing will get in our way. Drive taps into a more primal, foundational side of us.

If we are not considerate of our 'why', an extreme drive in only one of the 4 Pillars can develop at the expense of other areas in our life. If we are so driven to create wealth that we spend all our time at the office, our physical health and relationships will suffer. Consciously referencing our why and balance amongst the 4 Pillars is the key in creating a healthy drive.

Summary

Changing our habits is challenging. Yet, staying the same and doing nothing to improve is also challenging. Change is an exciting and inspiring process with the right knowledge and tools. Making small changes with the detail-oriented perspective of the 1% Rule and adapting the Kaizen approach to continual improvement supports our efforts to make consistent progress. Most importantly, understanding the nature of our minds and taking responsibility for the meaning we associate with failure can assist when things get difficult. Determining our 'why' serves as a meaningful basis for developing the healthy drive needed for success.

Before moving onto the next chapter, complete the activities below to develop a plan in creating new rituals and habits. It doesn't have to be the perfect plan, but we must start somewhere and we must start today.

Activities

1. What's a 1% change you can make today that would benefit you? For each of the pillars below list 1-2 small 1% changes that you can make and commit to doing today.

- Body
- Relationship
- Finances
- Mindset

2. Reflect on and list 3-4 points on why you are initiating changes in your rituals and habits in the first place? Are these reasons big enough to keep you going when things get tough? Perhaps write them on a sticky note and place it somewhere you can regularly see.

3. Where in your current life are you driven? Is it a healthy drive or is it impacting success in other pillars?

4. Reflect on your current values, what is important for you and the life you are creating? List your five most important values.

5. What does drive look like for you in each of the 4 Pillars? What actions would a driven person take in each of those areas?

Chapter 7 – Seeking Support

Successful people surround themselves with expertise. They go out of their way to listen and learn from masters of their crafts and do their best to integrate their knowledge and wisdom. It requires equal parts courage and humility to seek out people with experience and be open to their messages. Seeking support is vital in creating change as we acknowledge the challenges involved. Equipped with understanding, we can look for people with the right strategies and wisdom to support us in this process. The question is, do you see yourself as being successful in creating a life on your terms?

Each of us face our own individual set of challenges as we set goals and embrace change. A helping hand or guiding light during these times can mean the difference between sticking with it or giving up.

Why?

Seeking outside help through our challenges reflects our commitment to change and to our goals. When we invest financial resources into improving ourselves through attending a seminar or hiring a fitness professional, we demonstrate to ourselves that we value ourselves, our goal and are committed to achieve it.

The second benefit in opening to the influence of others is the different perspective they can offer. Regardless of who we seek support from or what we seek help for, an external opinion can open our minds to possibilities—to what we are capable of. Consider, for example, personal training. The quality of training a professional coach can provide far outweighs our own training knowledge. We will see results much faster and gain more knowledge regarding technique, nutrition, hydration, etc., through their knowledge and expertise than we would have discovered ourselves.

Likewise with a financial expert. Comprehending the myriad of investment choices available to us as well as tax and legal implications means it imperative to have a trusted advisor working in our corner. Obtaining knowledge about these opportunities as well as the practical accessibility of these opportunities can save us time, money and potentially much emotional stress and heartache.

The third benefit in seeking outside support is the emotional assistance they can provide. Making change can be a lonely process. Watching YouTube clips or listening to podcasts by people who faced great adversity and succeeded can fuel our motivation for another day or session. Having someone there, standing beside us as we progress can be the difference between success or failure.

Lone Wolf or Pack Mentality?

A place does exist for the lone wolf approach in undertaking change: where we face each challenge individually and work relentlessly through every obstacle we encounter. The mindset that 'I've got this' or 'I don't need any help' has its place. There are times when we simply have no one to ask for guidance and we must take a risk and initiate the next step. Some individuals thrive in this situation, where everything appears to be against them, and it is 100% up to them to keep moving forward. Being the lone wolf has its advantages—when we win, we own our victories; when we lose, we have no one to blame but ourselves as we pick ourselves up and start again. However, the lone wolf also misses out on some of the greatest advantages of belonging to a pack and may set themselves up for more challenges then necessary.

The mindset we are developing through mastering the 4 Pillars requires us to consider the advantages of creating our own pack, and to examine every 1% detail that will lead to success. By enlisting the help of a support crew or other like-minded individuals, we share the load together. We support their efforts as much as they support ours. We can schedule morning runs together or discuss financial strategies. There are many benefits available to us when we open ourselves up to create rituals and share our knowledge.

Finding the right people or resources for us in the areas of health, relationships, finance and mindset can mean that we establish many different 'packs.' Determining the right people or methods that work for us depend on many factors, such as the resources we have available, the time we have to invest and the ability to find the right people. Finding the right people to support us on this journey is perhaps the most challenging part, yet they do exist if we are creative in how we use our time and resources.

The concept of 'guru' may conjure up images of bearded Indian men dressed in saffron clothes espousing wisdom to all. The word guru translates to 'removal of darkness.' Our task is to find our own gurus to assist us in removing our own version of darkness. This darkness may be a lack of knowledge in a particular pillar, lack of emotional support or needing someone to hold us accountable for our actions. Whatever form it takes, developing our own 'pack' comprised of specific gurus can provide a catalyst for continued growth.

Resources to Help

Resourcefulness is the ultimate resource. To become creative with our thinking and our initiative and to seize opportunities when they arise is being resourceful. Action is always available to us. Taking the right action at the right time helps gather the support we need at a much faster rate than through trial and error by ourselves.

Attending seminars is one strategy in supporting our development. These events and seminars do not have to be expensive and with COVID, many are available globally and online. A recent shift in the marketing of some events makes them free of charge to encourage people to attend. When signing up for these events, we know there will be the inevitable 'sell' that occurs but there is always something to learn.

Attending seminars virtually or in person also creates opportunities to meet the right kind of people to further support us in our journey. Being in the same space with those who have also invested their time into a pursuit, enhances the possibility to connect with the right person. Perhaps we could be sitting beside a guru in the area that we are seeking support in? Or we may meet someone who can help us in any one of the 4 Pillars.

Attending events requires a clear intention of the outcome we desire. That outcome might be as diverse as the event itself, however, we need to be clear on our investment in time and what we hope to achieve. There have been many connections and relationships formed at such events as they draw together people who immediately share a common interest. Whatever the experience is, we have little to lose in attending.

It also takes courage to attend these events, particularly if single. Self-judgement and fear may inhibit our growth and prevent us from venturing out, particularly if knowledge is limited in a pillar. Courage is not the absence of fear. Courage is the ability to acknowledge fear and continue towards our desires. This courage is tested when placed in uncomfortable situations like attending a seminar. This is growth.

There are good lessons in putting ourselves in uncomfortable situations. Being vulnerable and open to opportunities allows unexpected breakthroughs. Mentors and inspiring people can be met in airports, gyms and even waiting rooms, just by opening conversations. I once met a multimillionaire who became my mentor just by initiating a conversation at the airport.

There should be no preconceived objectives from these conversations. The lesson is to always be open and ready. Taking a genuine interest in the person we are talking to and looking for ways we can help them creates great relationships and potentially leads to further contacts. Again, this reinforces the importance of maintaining high presentation. We never know who we might meet. Knowing we may only get one opportunity to make an impact, we must be prepared for that moment. It is always better to be prepared for the opportunity and for it not to arise than to have the opportunity and be unprepared.

Finally, hiring professionals to work with us supports our efforts to make progress. Professionals may be connected to any of the 4 Pillars and if they are good at what they do, we should see results quickly. Investments in working with personal trainers, financial advisers, relationship experts and psychologists are all valuable investments when they are the right ones for us and for our goals. Through some initial research, we can make sure they have the skills that we need.

Outsourcing

A word of caution. If we ask too many people to help, we risk trying to outsource our work in making change. We cannot allow professionals to assume our responsibilities. We must do the work.

We can work alongside others and even assist them towards their own desires but ultimately, we must take full responsibility for creating our own life. No individual can or should tell us what we must do to create our life. Accepting advice with gratitude and filtering that advice through our own intuition, experience and wisdom can help us make the decisions we need to make.

For the Love of Reading

Reading a diversity of books is probably the best and most cost-effective method for developing our own support. The accessibility of books means that we can literally read anywhere or anytime, and we do not have to go far to find them.

Reading for fifteen minutes a day equates to more than 90 minutes of reading a week and compounded over time impacts our brain development and thoughts. We can begin the process of reprogramming our mind through the books we read and knowledge we learn. Reading early in our day can inspire positive thoughts throughout the day and reading for a few minutes before sleep can assist with sleep quality. We can read on a train when going to work, on a plane when travelling overseas, during our lunch break or even while on the toilet!

The quality of the books you choose can have an enormous impact in learning the tools required to create a life on your terms. A book exists on every imaginable topic and demonstrates depth of character when speaking to people. Creating a book club within your circle of friends is great for relationships and moves conversations to a deeper level.

Summary

Developing ourselves requires many choices. Take some time now to think about the different avenues you could investigate to support yourself and the changes that you want to make. If you could create the ultimate support team, who would be in it and what role would they play? Would you enlist a trainer, a massage therapist or a relationship counselor? You already know what services you could benefit from and probably have some idea of where you could go to find out more information.

You might already know someone in that field and can barter an agreement to exchange services. It doesn't have to cost money if we are resourceful.

By seeking support, we demonstrate commitment in improving ourselves and become more accountable. With a focused and committed mindset, we can develop the courage needed to create our own pack, a community where we support and inspire each other. With support, the process of change is not only faster but more enjoyable.

Activities

1. Think about the different avenues you could investigate to support yourself and the changes you want to make. For each of the pillars below, list 2–3 external sources of help you can tap into to assist you and the work you are doing.

- Body
- Relationship
- Finances
- Mindset

2. Determine which friends may be interested in joining you on this journey in one area of the 4 Pillars. Perhaps an exercise buddy or relationship confidante? List support people for each of the 4 Pillars.

3. What expertise can you draw from successful people you already know in each of the 4 Pillars? What would you like to know from them and why? Do you have the courage to ask them for help?

4. Survey friends for recommendations on best books/podcasts to read/listen to in each of the 4 Pillars. Make a list of them and commit to purchasing/listening to at least one before the end of the month.

Chapter 8 – Maintaining Balance

As momentum grows in mastering the 4 Pillars and creating a life on our terms, so too does understanding balance. In the excitement of achievement, we can lose our sense of balance so we must cultivate this quality from the beginning.

What is meant by being balanced? At this moment in time, we are producing better results in one of the 4 Pillars than others. Our aim is to align all the pillars to the highest levels possible. A honed awareness of our sense of balance prevents us from over-investing in one pillar at the expense of another. It can also keep us on the right path when distractions arise.

Take a fitness fanatic and her concept of balance as an example. Her physique might be incredible, but does that mean she is a healthy, balanced human being? In order to achieve her great physique, she may have consumed many supplements, severely restricted her nutritional intake and perhaps even become 'addicted' to her physical appearance. Balanced? What about the person who is so committed in creating a 'happy' relationship that he will endure almost anything to keep his relationship together?

The examples also extend to the finance pillar. Consider the professionals who work long hours under a huge amount of pressure, to take home a big paycheck. While their bank balances and finances are in great shape, what about their physical health and the health of their relationships?

These are all extreme examples of an over-investment in one pillar at the expense of another, but they exist. We may already know people who resemble them. Chances are that if we speak with them about it, they will justify their actions. The fitness fanatic will say she feels good; the person in the dysfunctional relationship will say that it is better than being alone; and the professionals will say that they are working hard for their families.

All these reasons are valid but some lessons we can learn are from observing others and doing the opposite. We can admire their relentless drive and desire to create a life of meaning for them, yet we do not want to sacrifice success in one pillar at the expense of another.

Balance is critical as we experience success and see tangible results from our habits and rituals. Other people may notice our achievements and opportunities open to us.

It might be tempting to get carried away with our initial success. The more we master the 4 Pillars, the more distractions and opportunities unfold. Distractions in the form of other people, how we spend our time or even our developing ego all have the potential to sabotage our efforts.

Success can also be the enemy of progress. We may become 'infected' with the trappings of success and neglect the work that got us there. The discipline of continual improvement may be replaced with a sense of entitlement. Neglecting the 1% improvements, making us complacent and sloppy.

Balancing the excitement of success alongside opportunities arising from our progress is an unexpected challenge that can be hard to handle. When we begin to feel proud about our bodies or our financial situation improves, it is easy to develop an inflated opinion of ourselves and take short cuts with our habits and rituals. Our habits and rituals form the anchor that keeps us grounded and balanced in these times. Unless our foundation is balanced, any initial success will be short lived.

Reimagine Success

Stop for a moment and reflect on why you want to devote the time, energy and sacrifice in mastering the 4 Pillars and creating a life on your terms. Perhaps you feel something is missing and that you are not yet living your best life. Perhaps your health has declined over the years, or your mindset struggles when encountering challenges. Whatever your primary reason for wanting change, affirm that through your efforts, positive change can occur. Perhaps now is the time to reimagine or redefine success.

The attachment of happiness to an external achievement is a by-product of a society obsessed with ego and judgement, where we are encouraged to judge ourselves and others based on our car or our suburb. There are plenty of instances in our lives where we attached happiness to an external achievement only to recognise this excitement and happiness as fleeting. Perhaps the new car, new relationship or new job, once attained, wasn't quite so fulfilling after all.

Realising that we have two choices in how we address our emotions greatly impacts the quality of balance we bring to our lives. The first response is to set an even bigger goal or challenge for ourselves and relentlessly pursue that goal until we have achieved it. The second option is to enjoy and celebrate the success we have obtained, yet seek a deeper sense of satisfaction and happiness, unaffected by external achievements. Understanding that a certain level of excitement, energy and happiness automatically springs up when working on our goals can be our ticket to happiness. Appreciating this energy, growing our awareness, and enjoying this progress is the real measure of success. Continual progress is happiness.

I Want It All

Does that mean that we should relinquish the external pursuit of our desires in order to focus on internal peace and happiness? For some people, the answer to that question is yes; however, if you are anything like me, there is a good chance we have plenty of external desires to achieve as well. Why not have a fit and healthy body, amazing relationships, a great income and a positive mindset? I believe that the more we have, the more we can share. There is nothing great or noble in playing small, particularly when blessed with incredible talents to share. It is possible to achieve mastery of the 4 Pillars with the right foundations, positive mindset and consistent application in each of them.

The essential ingredient in balancing these desires is the understanding that our mind and ego will never be completely satisfied. Through awareness and acceptance of this relentless dissatisfaction, we can cultivate an appreciation for our journey and allow these desires to come to us.

Desire in and of itself is natural. Our experience of life has shaped and will continue to be shaped by our desires. We observe a beautiful car, and a rocket of desire is launched that we would like to feel the experience of driving that car. We witness a family sharing a meal together at the beach and another desire is launched. There are no limits to these desires that are continually being formed within us.

Relentlessly clinging to those desires as a perceived form of happiness will inevitably cause us to move out of balance or harmony from within. Harmony within is a state of alignment between our mind and heart and has nothing to do with our external circumstances. It's being able to draw inspiration from life's events, and consciously cultivate an expansive state of who we can be. This openness is free of judgement and attachment. It is the ultimate prize of life. Ironically, it is also the space where our greatest desires begin to unfold easily and naturally for us.

Balancing the Seesaw

Have you ever been on an old-fashioned seesaw, rarely seen in playgrounds nowadays? The ones where a person sits on either end of a beam that is balanced in the middle and both children swing up and down? I'm sure that for today's generation, this old piece of equipment would be considered pretty lame, but it provides a great reference point to consider when balancing all of the 4 Pillars.

This concept of the seesaw is the perfect analogy for maintaining balance when pursuing our desires. If we imagine one end of the beam to represent our energy, effort and unwavering commitment to achieving our desires and the other end to represent rest, relaxation and letting go, then we begin to see a clearer picture. Sometimes we need a little more energy and effort to form a new ritual, and other times we need to relax and allow change to happen for us. The key is to keep the seesaw balanced in a steady state while we are adjusting either end.

Throughout this process, our job is to observe each end of the seesaw and determine what side requires more effort. What keeps the beam balanced in the middle? Our focus. Yes, it's our ability to apply our attention and awareness consciously to our activities. Balancing the beam in one pillar can be a challenge yet applying the seesaw concept to all pillars can provide a useful reference point when determining what our next action should be. Sometimes the process of letting go and allowing nature to unfold for us can be the most challenging part. For high achievers, letting go can pose a real challenge. Letting go is not about giving up; it is surrendering our resistance to change. It means relinquishing control over the outcome. It means being prepared to let go of old habits to allow new ones to shape our lives in a different direction. Our bodies, relationships and even finances require us to develop the ability to let go.

The practical application of the seesaw concept within the 4 Pillars means that we have to determine when we need to invest more energy and commitment into one pillar and when we need to take a step back and let go in another. We may need to invest significantly more energy and time into creating a conscious ritual around our fitness or financial investments than our relationships. Or conversely, if our relationships are an area that we would like to improve, we'll take the uncomfortable step and introduce new actions. Only we know what activity needs greater emphasis and if it feels uncomfortable, then it is probably the right action for us. Why? Because growth occurs when we place ourselves in uncomfortable environments.

The term 'desirable difficulties', coined by psychologist Dr. Robert Bjork, states that effective learning occurs when the brain is exposed to challenges. When the learning process is messy, errors are high, and success is hard-won, long-term performance is improved. This means that by opening ourselves up to experience and accept the errors and mistakes we make, we have a greater chance of growing towards our goals.

Often, great things happen for us in times of rest when our conscious effort is minimal. Our body, for example can only recover, replenish and grow when resting at night. The action we take in developing our finances needs to be balanced in allowing time for our investments to grow. Our relationships also need time to evolve. Without letting go of this process, unnecessary suffering can result. Growth occurs once we have invested conscious effort in creating rituals and habits that place us in a position to receive these gifts. Remember it is AFTER we have done the work that rest and letting go can occur, not before!

The concept of the seesaw is loosely based on the interpretation of the three gunas as written by Eddie Stern in *One Simple Thing* (2020). Represented within yoga, the gunas represent three constituents of our mind: rajas—effort, tamas—rest and sattva—knowing. Through this interpretation of the gunas, it is said that all things manifest in the world and applying our focus in balancing our effort with appropriate amounts of rest or letting go can be the catalyst for big things to occur.

Summary

Finding balance among the 4 Pillars is a challenge. It can be even more challenging to maintain balance when we experience success and new opportunities emerge. It is possible to create an outstanding life on our terms where each pillar of health, relationship, finance and mindset is operating at its absolute potential. Desires are continually being formed within us through the experiences we have and the events that we witness. Maintaining an overall sense of balance or harmony keeps us in the game and progressing forward.

Activities

1. What does balance mean to you, and would you consider yourself a 'balanced' person at this time? Are there areas in your life that you feel are more balanced than others?

2. In each area of Health, Relationships, Finances and Mindset determine how much time you have to invest in them on a daily basis. What pillars require a greater investment in time to balance out the remaining pillars?

3. What people do you know who you consider balanced in one of the 4 Pillars? Could you ask them for any advice or guidance that you can apply in your own life?

4. What does a balanced day look like for you? What actions can you take to bring balance into your daily life?

PART II

The journey of a thousand miles begins with a single step.
– Lao Tzu

ACTION Time

Now is the time to witness the 4 Pillars in action and create a life reflective of your desires and the person you are choosing to become. How necessary it is to have rituals and habits when setbacks occur, and uncertainty is high? How can a healthy body support us when we contend with disappointment? How much more supportive is a network of solid friendships when it is based on mutual values and will bolster us when we're struggling?

To emphasise the application of the 4 Pillars, Part II is an invitation to start your journey now, together with me, in creating a life on your terms. Together, we can progress through life-changing decisions and undertake substantial, step by step change.

My hope for this section is that we can walk together and strategize as we confront and overcome physical, mental and emotional challenges. We can see firsthand how our daily rituals and choices support our progress, even when it appears none is made.

Finally, my mission is to inspire you. Although the challenges and obstacles presented to us are tough, cultivating a positive internal mindset helps us win each day. With the right mindset, we can appreciate the tough moments, knowing they will pass as well as teach us something about ourselves and our ability to manage our resources. Through these experiences, we learn so much about ourselves, our fears and our unlimited potential. We find joy and fulfillment in making a commitment to improving ourselves through one small action at a time.

Success in life is rarely won or lost in a single moment. Substantial achievement results from many small moments, lessons and decisions from our action or inaction. This moment, right now, presents the opportunity for us to begin the process of change in mastering the 4 Pillars.

Week 1: Creating a Strong Foundation

The first step towards getting somewhere is to decide
that you are not going to stay where you are.
– J.P. Morgan, Financier

What is holding you back from creating a life on your terms?
How would it feel to create a life where you determine how
you spend your time? Week One of this eight-week program
is designed to acknowledge the past and plan for a new future:
one where you actively take control of living the life that you
have defined as a success.

In Part I of this book, activities were selected to provide
clarity around the decisions you need to make. Now is the
time to implement those plans. It's time to take control of
the change process and use your insight to create the life you
desire. Most importantly, this journey creates a foundation for
change where YOU control the process, where your actions
are aligned with your internal belief system and processes are
in place to support you during challenges.

Only eight weeks to create the perfect life on your terms?
No.

It takes eight weeks to shift the current course of your life
and begin falling in love with the process of change, a process
that up until now, you may not have consciously navigated. With
the right amount of enthusiasm, practice and compassion, we
can begin to master the process of change, enabling our desires
to unfold.

Defining Your Purpose

Why do you want to take the actions and risks necessary to lead
a better life, particularly when society and the world around us

values security and comfort? Burning desires may be enough for some to scale great heights but for others, defining a higher purpose may be the spark that ignites sustainable action.

Defining a higher purpose requires us to analyze our strengths, values and beliefs. It requires deep reflection into our nature and developing an understanding of who we are and what we are called to do. Accurately summarized in Viktor Frankl's book *Man's Search for Meaning* (1946) about his experience in Auschwitz, a Nazi death camp, if we can find meaning from our struggles than we can endure almost any challenge. Our meaning may not always be glamorous, but once we align with it, our actions are directed from a deeper place as we grow more resilient.

Our contribution to our community lies at the very center of defining our purpose and determining how best we can use our talents and skills for the betterment of others. For some, this higher purpose may be in the form of pursuing sporting excellence or musical mastery. For others, such as Blessed Mother Theresa of Kolkata, it may be a calling to work with the disadvantaged, the disenfranchised and the dying. Regardless of the style of our contribution, once we align our actions with our central purpose, our lives begin to shine.

Simon Chokoisky in *The 5 Dharma Types* (2014) wrote of five different destinies that encapsulate our purpose on earth. These dharma types, duties or callings are unique to each person and once aligned with our predominant dharma, our actions provide us with a greater sense of meaning. The five dharmas: educator, warrior, merchant, labourer and outsider all fulfill different roles within society and contribute in their own unique ways.

Regardless of the nature of our employment, we can still exhibit these attributes. For example, an educator may not always be a schoolteacher. Individuals with the predominant dharma of educator will naturally enjoy educating people in any role they undertake. Educators can express their calling through writing, healthcare, training, or any other method that allows them to express their dharma.

Once we understand and develop an appreciation of our dharma, we can then shape our actions according to our higher purpose. A lawyer may find fulfillment of her warrior dharma through defending environmental destruction in the court system. The labourer may feel peace in his contribution of constructing beautiful buildings or working with his hands as a craftsperson. A good indicator of what our dharma is can be found in growing our awareness of what activities inspire us with energy.

Attitude Determines Altitude

Our attitude and commitment in defining our higher purpose provides a strong foundation for change. Once clear on our purpose, our attitude towards the change process becomes easier. For example, if we determine that being the best possible father for our children provides meaning for us, we have a reason for developing a positive attitude towards a new health regime. Attitude shapes our interpretation of life events. With a positive, determined and committed attitude, failures become obstacles we will overcome along the path to success.

To gain the most from this program, three cornerstones of attitude should be reflected upon:

- Show Up: Showing up means we are fully committed to whatever activity we are doing. It means we bring energy, enthusiasm and a clear sense of purpose to all that we do. Showing up means we are engaged, present and willing to lay it all on the line in the achievement of our goal.

- Try Something New: Trying something new is opening ourselves up to new experiences. It means we accept the setbacks that may occur, yet we are still prepared to take risks. Trying something new is looking for new ways to do activities we have always done.

- Be Consistent: Being consistent is taking the attitude of 'showing up' and 'trying something new' and bringing a level of commitment for a sustained period. It's the ability to continue to believe that the process of change will work for us even if we do not see immediate results. Being consistent is the foundation for the compound effect.

A New Mindset

Let's begin with the ultimate tool at our disposal for creating this change process: our mindset. Up until now, our mind has largely created the world we experience. Through our interpretation and imagination of the world we experience around us, we formed beliefs about our capacity to create the life we desire. From our health, relationships and finances our mindset initiates the actions that produces the results we experience. The mind is the ultimate creation tool. It has served us well, bringing us to this junction but it may need an upgrade in thinking and beliefs. Like a computer system constantly requiring software updates, our mindset also requires continual development.

Prominent psychologist and best-selling author, Dr. Carol Dweck explored two varying mindsets that impact our ability to grow and undertake change. In her book, *mindset* (2017) the concepts of fixed and growth mindsets are presented as two opposing forces impacting our ability to learn and change. People with a predominantly fixed mindset view intelligence, knowledge and character as static, and devote their time and energy in protecting this belief. The notion of the gifted athlete or the natural musician fits in with this perception as examples of people simply born with set characteristics rather than choosing them. A fixed mindset perceives change as a threat and identifies external results as a reflection of character. If my partner leaves me, there must be something wrong with me is another example of the fixed mindset in action.

Alternatively, a growth mindset is established towards purposeful engagement with a focus on continual development. Individuals with a growth mindset welcome change and understand that failure does not define them. A financial setback is seen as an opportunity to identify new strategies for improvement towards the goal. In a growth mindset, curiosity and a sustained work ethic create opportunities for learning, naturally leading to improved results. More importantly, Dr. Dweck presents the notion that a growth mindset is learnable at any age with the right awareness and attitude.

Throughout the next eight weeks, our attitude towards change will test our mindset. Are we working with a growth or fixed mindset in the areas of health, relationships and finances? Predictably, we can be a mixture of both mindsets at different times and in different areas. We might be open to the growth mindset when undertaking changes in our health yet fixed in our relationships.

Understanding our mindset towards change will impact our enthusiasm, energy and ultimately our results. Adopting a growth mindset from the beginning gives us the best chance of success.

Week 1 Activity

Let's make peace with where we are in our life right now.

Week 1 activity is purchasing a journal for use in setting intentions and reflections for the next eight weeks. A journal to acknowledge our journey to this point in time and to prepare a new way to approach change.

To begin using this journal, plan time out of your daily routine. Take a hike in the woods to clear the lungs, a long walk by the beach, or any special place away from people. Nature has the ability to simplify our thinking and create space. Become aware of your dominant thoughts as you walk and allow at least a couple of hours for this process. How you begin any activity defines the quality that you produce. To create a life on your terms, you must honor this ritual by bringing your best attitude.

Throughout the first half of your hike, reflect on the things you are grateful for in each of 4 Pillars. Try to feel and experience this gratefulness. At some point along your journey, stop and observe the environment you are in. Express gratitude that you are alive here and now. Fill your lungs with clear air as you record in your journal these specific areas of gratitude from your health, relationships, finances and mindset.

If you're not sure where to start, first consider your body. Perhaps you're grateful for your health. If you're single, consider this a time to develop self-love. Challenges with finances may provide clarity in what you desire or gratitude for taking ownership of your mindset. There is no better place to begin the journey of creating a life on our terms than from a place of gratitude.

Now as you move further along in your journey into nature and self-inquiry, consider small changes in each of the 4 Pillars you would like to implement in your life. Try to select changes that excite and motivate you. Create goals around feelings and emotions, such as determining ways to create more energy and vitality forces. Examples include developing a positive attitude toward exercising/nutrition, actively listening when talking with your partner, feeling enjoyment investing your money and journaling your thoughts at the end of each day. These internal goals provide 100% control over the outcome and are far more achievable than many external goals we set.

External goals provide an opportunity to practice and test the development of our internal goals. A more positive attitude toward exercise may result in you exercising for 30 minutes each day. Actively listening to your partner will allow you to compliment them in a more specific manner. Feeling enjoyment when investing money will help excite and motivate you to save more. Journaling your thoughts is a productive method for developing awareness of our internal dialogue. A balanced approach between internal and external goals provides a good starting point.

Remember the Kaizen principle and the 1% Rule for improvement in selecting your goals. Ask how you would feel after imbedding this change into your being. Try to envision what you would look like and how you would act. Answering these questions ignites a deeper part of our consciousness, further drawing us towards new beliefs and actions.

As a final act before completing your time in nature, write a letter to yourself. This reflective letter draws together the gratitude you are currently experiencing as well as setting new intentions for the future. A hand-written letter is best, as it's a powerful emotional focus tool, connecting our visual and kinesthetic senses with our internal thoughts. In seeing words expressed on paper, our mind has an increased ability to believe those words, positively impacting our emotions.

Keep this letter close by and continue to journal your thoughts over the next eight weeks. Place the letter somewhere you can regularly see it or carry it with you when you are out. Feel the power in creating new intentions and be drawn towards the desires you have set.

This is the priority action item for the first week and provides a foundation for our decisions to flow.

Summary of Journaling Activity

- Reflect and record specific areas of gratefulness for each Pillar
- Create four internal goals from each of the 4 Pillars
- Determine an external goal that will enable clear action in alignment with your internal goal
- Record your anticipated feelings once these goals are accomplished
- Write a letter to yourself setting intentions and cementing your commitment to the next eight weeks.
- Place your new goals and intentions somewhere you can regularly review them

Making a Decision

Every action begins with an internal decision that impacts our external environment from the ripples it causes and the results we experience. The meaning of the word decision comes from the Latin root word of 'cis' meaning to 'cut' or 'kill.' In making a decision, we are literally cutting off other possibilities with our choice.

In journaling our thoughts by writing a reflective letter to ourselves, we are committing to cut off alternative actions that prevent us from achieving the desires we hold. We take a stand and begin to make decisions from that standpoint. With this understanding, clarity is gained and focus is enhanced. We now have a place to return each time we encounter resistance and a point of reference when faced with challenges.

Cleanliness is Godliness

Throughout the rest of the week, devote time to 'clearing' your backyard in each of the 4 Pillars. Seek the professional assistance of those who can help clear the challenges in each of the 4 Pillars as a demonstration of your commitment through your actions. This may entail a health examination or consultation with a financial adviser. It may include seeking relationship guidance from a close friend or downloading a meditation app. In the initial stages of change, we want to do everything we can to clear away debris that may slow our progress.

We can express the notion of clearing away old patterns across all areas of our lives as well. Clearing our closet of old clothes or furniture and donating these items to charity has the added benefit of assisting us to feel good as well as contributing to others in need. We can also clear our pantry of food that no longer support the person we are choosing to become. Physically cleaning our home, our possessions and our relationships opens the doorway for new habits to enter.

A clean environment cleans our internal mindset. Unwanted negativity, laziness and self-deprecation festers in an unclean environment. When we are our surrounded by untidiness, disorder and general clutter, our mindset is impacted in a negative way.

Cleanliness also enhances self-satisfaction. Feeling self-satisfied in performing the small acts of cleanliness promotes awareness and appreciation. We do not need many possessions or a big house to grow this sense of satisfaction. It can easily come to us through placing our efforts in performing the small tasks required to keep our surroundings clean.

Weekly Reflections

Week One is the foundation for the coming weeks. From a strong foundation, clear decisions are made with energy and purpose. A foundation based on gratitude and acceptance for our present gifts provide a stable base to begin crafting a new life. Every day is a miracle and conditioning ourselves to witness this miracle sharpens our desire to make the most of it.

Throughout the next eight weeks, we will continually return to this feel good, grateful place when faced with challenges. We will reflect upon our attitude and mindset and take time to attend to the small details in maintaining cleanliness in our life.

Activities

1. What is your purpose and what provides meaning for your actions? How can you link your desire for change to a larger contribution to your community or society?

2. Reflect on your current attitude toward change. What has prevented you from showing up, trying something new and being consistent in the past?

3. Assess your mindset. Are you a growth or closed mindset person? How can you develop more awareness around this?

4. Create a list of 3-5 immediate tasks that you can perform this week to 'clean' your life. Perhaps there are some parts you know require cleaning that you have avoided up until now.

6. Are you clear on your values? Do your values align with your goals?

Use your newly purchased journal to record your thoughts on potential fears for the next eight weeks.

Week 2: Establishing New Habits

> We are what we repeatedly do.
> Excellence, then, is not an act, but a habit.
> – Aristotle, Greek Philosopher

For Week Two, we'll implement our new habits and rituals. We will build on the activities from the first week and develop strategies to incorporate new actions into our daily lives. We are cultivating a foundation, purpose and positive attitude and this week we will action them. We have initiated the clearing of unnecessary resistance from our lives. Adjustment of our previous habits allows us to incorporate new rituals, and these efforts are supported by organizational planning.

When, Where, How?

Planning at the beginning of the week makes our transition easier. Determining when, where and how we will perform our new rituals can resolve potential problems before they emerge. With our 'why' determined during our work in Week One, the remaining details are logistical. Planning and attention to detail will foster our success.

This week, we can start with clear communication of our plans to those who will be impacted by them. Support from others is critical to the ongoing success of any change process, so take the time to sit down and explain your new habits, rituals and your motivation. Relationships underpin much of our happiness and others can become fearful and or negative if they hold a fixed mindset and perceive us as changing in ways they don't understand. Our loved ones deserve an explanation for this effort. Enlisting their support can alleviate their concerns, hold us accountable and serve as inspiration for their own journey.

In planning our 'when, where and how' at the beginning of this and subsequent weeks, we are in control of the change process. We are using our journals to pencil in a time and place for our activities to create confidence that these events will occur. We may even have back-up plans when challenges arise.

Clarity and precision around our activities for the week provides certainty in completing them. 'Getting into shape' or 'learning to cook' is too vague and will impact our motivation as we cannot clearly see when we have completed them. A sense of accomplishment comes from the clear completion of our goals and this clarity occurs in the planning stage.

Early morning is a good time to execute our plans while our heads are clear and distractions are few. Our energy and enthusiasm are strong in the morning and we can complete new rituals with vigour. To be 100% prepared for our morning rituals, we should consider our evening routines.

Evening Routines

Research from Consumer Reports on consumerreports.org indicates that up to 80% of Americans report problems with sleep at least once a week, impacting their health, happiness and performance. Sleep statistics from the Center of Disease Control and Prevention show that up to 35% of Americans don't get the recommended seven hours of sleep each night and almost 97% of teenagers are classified as sleep deprived. As a society, we have gone from an average of nine hours of sleep per night to less than seven in just over a century. From fatigue and an increased risk of obesity to anxiety and stress-related illnesses, sleep deprivation affects every area of our lives.

With many competing distractions, it can be a challenge to remain physically in bed for eight to nine hours per night. Fifty percent of Americans report difficulty in staying asleep, waking at least once per night and struggling to get back to sleep again. At best, this can be frustrating, at its worst, insomnia can increase anxiety and stress related disorders. Let's consider two aspects of our sleep patterns: firstly, the length of our sleep; and secondly, its quality. Planning and adhering to bedtime rituals assist the body's need to unwind and relax before falling asleep.

Our evening rituals should consider several variables, including the length of time from our last meal, technology interaction and what time we would like to rise in the morning. We also need to know the amount of hours we require to function at our best.

First, determine what time you would like to get out of bed in the morning and work backwards from there. If you decide to rise by 6a.m., then in order to get the recommended seven-eight hours of sleep, be in bed by 10-11 p.m.

There are no rules for determining this process and timing will fluctuate but having a good idea of what time we would like to be in bed assists our decision making. If we know the Netflix show we are watching will finish later then the time we've set for bed, than we have a decision to make and as stated, these little decisions become the life we create.

In developing consistency with the time we go to sleep, our body naturally begins to release sleep hormones such as melatonin. We begin to feel tired at the same time each night. Our sleep quality and the energy we have to plan and complete our new rituals largely depends on the quality of our evening rituals.

Aside from mandatory routine tasks like brushing our teeth, developing a ritual to slow the physical and mental side of the body down assist in quickly falling asleep. Nothing is more frustrating that lying awake in bed, planning, or thinking about tomorrow. Small actions such as turning off screens for our phones, computers and televisions and reducing unnecessary noise allow the brain to decompress. Physical activities such as taking a slow walk after dinner, stretching, or meditating also aid digestion and calm the mind.

Mastery of the 4 Pillars is the result of unwavering commitment in performing the 1% activities. As famous American Football coach Vince Lombardi said, 'To achieve success, whatever the job you have, you must pay a price.' Developing an evening routine is a small price to pay in establishing a strong start to your day.

Other strategies include sitting still for an evening meditation or reflecting on our thoughts and mindset in our journal. Reading an uplifting book or having a quiet cup of herbal tea are other alternatives. Spending uninterrupted time with your partner is an effective way to end a day and invest in your relationship at the same time.

As a final practice, try lying completely still on the floor, resting your body and softening your energy. This 'earthing' or grounding practice helps in preparing for the transition from wakefulness to sleep. Earthing is usually associated with walking barefoot outside in connecting the body to the natural environment. The same concept applies in lying on the floor and connecting your body to a hard, flat surface. Eric Muller, et al., published an article in *Frontiers in Physiology* highlighting benefits of such practice including improved sleep, reduced inflammation and a reduction in muscle soreness. Five minutes of muscle relaxation and mental rest on a hard surface can be the best transition before getting into bed.

For a final strategy to prepare the mind for the next day, focus your thoughts on positive events that occurred throughout the day. Reflecting on one area within each of the 4 Pillars with gratitude conditions the mind to appreciate and anticipate the positives each day. The more we look for and emphasize these positive events in our lives, the more they grow.

Procrastination

Procrastination has the potential to derail our best efforts in completing our rituals and this week is a good time to address it. We can have the best reasons and plans to change, yet if there is still resistance towards performing these new rituals than it is wise to explore possible barriers. Even if our new rituals are the simplest of activities, procrastination can impact our motivation.

Procrastination is the voluntary delaying of intended tasks we know we can easily complete yet for whatever reason, we fail to undertake. Research from the Carleton University Procrastination Research Group identifies that procrastination impacts our physical and mental wellbeing and can include delaying simple tasks such as writing an email or changing an ink cartridge.

If we identify a tendency to procrastinate from past experiences in any area of the 4 Pillars, now is the time to create a positive approach with procrastination. Timothy Pychyl, a psychology professor at Carleton University in Ottawa and author of *Solving the Procrastination Puzzle* (2013) suggests immediate action the next time we encounter this resistance. When we complete a task without thinking about it for long, the attention remains on action rather than emotional resistance. Once we begin taking action, Pychyl states the process of completing the task becomes easier.

Another strategy for tackling procrastination is the two-minute rule by David Allen, American productivity consultant and author of *Getting Things Done* (2019). Allen states that if the activity will take fewer than two minutes, it is more effective to dive in and complete the task than to spend the energy avoiding it. Making the phone call, sending the message, or getting out the door for the early morning jog are the key challenges for most procrastinators. Planning makes this transition from thinking to action easier. Have the jogging shoes and clothes laid out the evening before the run to move into action before there is a chance to procrastinate.

Initial Success

Often the universe will assist us in our first few decisions throughout the week and we'll believe that the journey ahead will be quick and easy. We'll have breakthroughs in our health, relationships or finances and believe everything will continue to flow. Just as we begin to develop confidence through those first tentative steps of actions, we might also encounter a test or series of tests. These challenges are necessary for our evolution. How we confront each one and the lessons we experience can support our growth and resilience if we let them.

Success never happens overnight. No matter how much we may want quick success, we have to be prepared for relentless effort. Getting up an extra 30 minutes at the start of the day for this work is a challenge. It is also fulfilling and satisfying in another, deeper way. Once we're up, these positive efforts will stick with us throughout the day. Crafting and cultivating new rituals, turning them into habits and seeking outside help assists us in reaching our greater goals.

Don't be disheartened if you doubt the effectiveness of your goals for this week. Creating a compelling vision for your life takes time. Determining what that vision is and the associated actions often occur through trial and error. Thomas Edison made between 1,000 to 6,000 attempts before he invented the lightbulb. Through each failed attempt, he learned a little more and progressed a little closer to his goal.

Alignment with Values

Reflecting on our chosen activities for the week ahead and their alignment with our values confirms we are making the right decisions. The decisions we make must be right for us, not for the sake of others.

Edith Eger, Auschwitz survivor and psychologist discusses in her book, *The Choice* (2018), four simple questions she asks her clients in determining the choices they can make in moving beyond trauma,

- What do you want?
- Who wants it?
- What are you going to do about it?
- When?

While the questions look easy to complete on paper, the activity requires a deep reflection on who we are and what direction we are choosing to move in. Have you thought deeply as to what you truly want and where you see yourself five years from now? Are these choices in complete alignment with your values or are you living someone else's life? Perhaps you have found yourself living a life determined from the environment you grew up in or the people you associate with. If you could do anything, what would it be? Are you brave enough to do something about it and act towards creating it?

Our values underpin our thoughts, which in turn, create our beliefs and ultimately our actions. If the tasks we assign ourselves align with our values, then they are easier to perform. If we value having great relationships, then taking the time to send a message or organize a Zoom meeting with a friend will be easier than if other values rank higher on our priority list.

If an activity on our list is important to us, yet conflicts with our values, the challenge is to find a way to make it enjoyable. If eating healthier is a new ritual we would like to create, but don't enjoy the process of cooking, then creatively looking for ways to enjoy the cooking process may make things easier. Getting together with friends once a week for a 'cook-off' of healthy food or purchasing a subscription from a delivery service of healthy ingredients and recipes are creative options to enjoy this activity.

Weekly Reflection

The intention for Week Two is to begin living our new rituals through planning and developing strategies to overcome resistance or procrastination. Through this process, we develop clarity around our goals and communicate our changes to the people most impacted by them.

Our evening routines provide a structure for calming the body and mind and for the transition from wakefulness to sleep. The quality of our evening routines lay the foundation for our energy and enthusiasm in completing our goals the next morning. Success in achieving our goals will come from alignment with values and creating small rituals that can support the person we are choosing to become.

Activities

1. Reflect on your week and list five successes from planning and implementing your new rituals. How did you feel when completing them? What part of the process did you enjoy?

2. How did these successes impact your mindset for the rest of the day?

3. List your evening routine for the week. Did it impact your performance in completing your new rituals?

4. Identify enhancements and specific actions you can take to improve your evening routine. Can you adapt your plans and strategies in any way to enhance your outcomes?

5. Identify your values for each of the 4 Pillars in your journal and the importance in living those values.

6. Throughout your day, ask yourself these questions,

- What do I want?
- Who wants it?
- What am I going to do about it?
- When?

Week 3: Taking Risks

Only those who risk going too far
can possibly find out how far
one can go.
– T.S. Eliot, poet

Everything in life involves risk, from our relationships and financial affairs to driving a car. Sometimes not taking a risk poses an even bigger risk. If we don't take a risk and move our bodies, for example, it will deteriorate.

This week, we will develop our risk-taking 'muscle.' We will use our new rituals and habits as the basis for increasing our risk-taking activities. Why? Because taking risks develops our growth mindset, expands our comfort zone and presents new opportunities for change.

Risk-taking is not something that comes naturally for most of us and like any skill we want to develop, we begin with little steps, or micro risks. If we start with small risks where the consequences for failure are small, we can grow into taking larger risks equalling larger results.

New Risks

For each of our four new rituals devised from each of the 4 Pillars in Week One, Week Three's activity is to plan to take a new risk associated with that ritual. It could be working out in slightly different way, asking a friend out to lunch or setting up a savings account for our finances. Once again, the process of growing more at ease with setting risks and working outside our comfort zone is the real challenge, not the activities themselves. Progress comes from developing our skills of experiencing fear and uncertainty, and still proceeding with our objectives.

Decisions and planning are the first step, followed by action. A little fear and nervous excitement in determining what our actions will be indicates we are on the right track. The balance between excitement and fear propels us further forward. The excitement of accomplishing a goal we set for ourselves combined with the potential for failure drives us. Getting this balance right requires reflection and unwavering commitment.

If we have chosen activities that are not too threatening, the fear of setback should be minimal. If our fear factor is high, perhaps we should dial it down with an easier task. Remember, the amygdala is easily triggered when taking on new activities and we want to enjoy taking these risks. We can also reward ourselves when we take action. Choose simple rewards, as eventually, we want to get hooked on the excitement of taking risks rather than the reward. An initial, external positive reward like purchasing a new yoga mat or running sneakers, planning a date night at that fancy restaurant you've been eyeing, or booking in for a massage is still a good way to acknowledge the action we have taken. Remember to reward the action not the outcome.

Just like our tasks for Week Two, be specific on the details of the risk you want to take. Along with the risk itself, pencil in a time and place for this to occur. This level of detail— the when and where—holds us accountable. It's easy to make excuses when the unexpected occurs and our plans are delayed. And something will come up, probably just as we are about to act. We might wake up to rain when we have scheduled a training session, or someone will interrupt as we engage in a deep conversation. Whatever the unforeseen event is, be prepared to pivot with a predetermined back-up plan to stay focused.

A subtle trick the mind might play during these moments is to convince us to delay our risk-taking action. The thought will arise that 'perhaps this is not the right time' and we will consider stalling. As the mind tries to protect us from failure, it uses its intimate knowledge of our fears to undermine the action. Remember the mind seeks comfort and security.

Many will listen to this inner conversation and delay the action until a 'better time.' The attitude of 'When this happens, I will...' prevents them from taking the action necessary for positive change. Delaying action stalls our progress. By increasing our awareness around this inner dialogue, we begin the process of deliberate practice.

Deliberate Practice

The concept of 10,000 hours of practice to master a skill is not new. This number derives from the work of psychologist Anders Ericsson and others who released an academic paper in 1993. Their research found that people achieving at the highest level in musical performance had accumulated approximately 10,000 hours or two and a half hours of effort each day for 10 years.

Consider that for a moment. They put two and a half hours of effort a day for 10 years before they reached that level of mastery where they were recognized by their peers as experts. Most people don't realize that within the same paper, their evidence clearly indicated that high achievers are always made and are not born. They persisted in their craft long after the 'gifted' gave up and it enabled them to achieve a level of mastery that for most people, appeared abnormal. Natural ability only takes us so far in achieving success in each of the 4 Pillars, and persistence makes all the difference.

Does that mean we have to spend 10 years to achieve our desires of mastery in each of the 4 Pillars? Perhaps not. Also, within the same paper, Ericsson noted that many of the people in his study had accumulated 'substantially fewer' than 10,000 hours of practice. He noted that the quality of the practice was the difference and those who were involved in deliberate practice achieved results faster than those that didn't.

The term deliberate practice (DP) refers to the specific and sustained effort to focus on things that we can't do well. DP requires 'struggle, sacrifice and honest, often painful self-assessment.' In other words, it requires persistence. DP continually places us outside of our comfort zones as we seek challenging experiences. This work dovetails with that of Robert Bjork and the notion of 'desirable difficulties,' which means the best learning and growth occurs when we consciously choose the high road or hidden path.

Everyone who has achieved big desires has either knowingly or unknowingly chosen this path. From NASA astronauts to basketball legends such as Michael Jordan, individuals who are out there living life on their terms practice DP every day. DP trumps age, passion, intelligence, money and genes. By taking deliberate action that makes us feel slightly uncomfortable, we grow in confidence to take on bigger actions, naturally leading to bigger results.

Is there supplemental knowledge you need to acquire to deliberately practice your risk-taking skills in areas of the 4 Pillars? Is there some external support you can call on for assistance in this area?

Be specific and remember that our micro risks should feel so small that practicing DP is likely to result in success. A micro risk could be as simple as saying good morning to all your work colleagues when you enter the office tomorrow or leaving a note of gratitude for your partner. Remember that the fight, flight or freeze system of the brain, the amygdala, is easily triggered when taking on large risks, so keep it simple. Going for a morning walk, creating a money jar or listening to a five-minute meditation app are additional examples that most of us can complete without fear or anxiety. DP teaches us that we can continually improve and eventually master our risk-taking skills if we bring the right amount of energy and enthusiasm for a sustained period.

Keep Moving Forward

Negative self-talk and judgement are obstacles that can impact our risk-taking progress. They require analysis and understanding. The self-imposed judgement we place on ourselves prevents us from taking on any risks and challenges that we may perceive as dangerous. Irrational fear of what people think and what we think about ourselves, means that we unconsciously live a smaller life than what we are capable of.

Negative self-talk can become a self-fulfilling prophecy. If we constantly tell ourselves we can't do something, we won't ever be able to do it. The language we use to describe and frame events is critical.

This negative self-talk can be triggered even when taking on micro risks. We cannot fuel this negative self-talk, otherwise, it prevents us from taking action. The Cherokee story of the 'Two Wolves' is a reminder of the internal battle between positive and negative forces.

> One evening, a grandfather spoke to his grandson
> about the battle that goes on inside people's heads.
> He said, "It is as if there are two wolves inside of us.
> One wolf is good and does no harm. He is joy, peace,
> strength, hope, serenity, kindness, compassion and love.
> He lives in harmony with all around him and does not
> take offense when no offense was intended. He will
> only fight when it is right to do so, and in the right
> way. But the other wolf is anger, greed, jealousy, sorrow,
> anxiety, self-pity, resentment and fear. The littlest thing
> sets him into a fit of anger. He fights everyone, all the
> time, for no reason. He cannot think because his anger

and fear are so great. Sometimes it is hard to live with these two wolves inside us, for both of them seek to dominate our spirit."

The grandson thought for a moment and asked, "Which one wins, Grandfather?"

The grandfather smiled and replied, "The one you feed."

Fortunately, when we develop awareness of our self-talk, we can see how it impacts us and the life we create. Focusing on positive self-talk, eating nutritious food and many other rituals builds strength for our 'good' wolf. Physical health and wellbeing impact our self-talk. If our body is in top shape by maintaining consistency in practicing our rituals, our inner voice and mindset will be positive.

Pivoting vs. Persistence

Reflecting on your risk-taking challenges can reveal many insights. Did the execution of your risk go according to plan? During these risk-taking moments, how did you feel? What was your thinking? Did you change your approach to get the desired outcome?

Perhaps in modifying your gym program, you allowed for extra recovery. Or maybe you improvised with a different set of questions when out to lunch with a friend. It doesn't matter how we modify or change our approach when taking risks, it's our increasing ability to pivot when faced with uncertain outcomes that is the win. When taking risks, observing information and adapting our approach are the keys to achieving successful outcomes. Adaptability only develops through risk-taking moments. The deliberate practice of entering these situations and pivoting whilst in the middle of change or even chaos is growth and builds pathways to a better life.

Fire of Desire

Within each of us exists a desire to live a better life, represented as an internal fire, the 'fire of desire.' Some people develop a raging, unstoppable fire that destroys everyone and everything in their path. Ultimately, this raging fire destroys them through obsessiveness, aggressiveness and attachment. While other people have a small hidden flame, fearful of sharing this gift for a multitude of reasons.

If we can acknowledge that our own desires are a gift from a higher source, we can begin to cultivate them in a more positive manner. The works of Warren Buffet and Bill Gates are examples of people who have acquired great wealth and have used that wealth for the benefit of millions of people. By linking our desires to noble pursuits, such as inspiring others, contributing to society or supporting environmental care, we can shape meaning and purpose behind each action we take, positively drawing energy to help us continue to take risks.

It is up to us to determine what our gifts are and how we draw them out into the world. Training the mind through positive self-talk phrases such as, 'The more I have, the more I can give,' and 'There is no inspiration in playing small for others' sake,' can assist in developing the courage needed to uncover what these desires are.

In Napoleon Hill's famous 1937 book, *Think and Grow Rich*, success in any domain begins with developing a burning desire or hunger. Through this desire, we pursue our goals with passion, energy, intense enthusiasm and pride. We find enjoyment in what we are doing along with fulfilment and alignment with our highest self. Our amygdala is positively activated. Positive emotions and feelings of wellbeing flood the body. Our prefrontal cortex, responsible for higher-order cognitive thinking and actions, is also activated. Our decisions are guided with definitive purpose and we have the passion, resilience and energy we need to sustain us when we are challenged.

Weekly Reflection

Changes are occurring within and around us every week. On the surface, everything may still look the same and progress may be slow. Do not be discouraged. We may not yet see substantial changes in our health, relationships, finances, or mindset from our work over the last three weeks and that is OK. We are developing and growing a foundation for a new being and reality.

We are developing the mindset that accepts the challenge of taking risks in the four areas of life that have the greatest impact on our quality of life. Improvements in our health, relationships, finances and mindset all require some risk-taking. These risks can be small, calculated and non-threatening. Over time they will build, like the fire of desire we are carefully cultivating within us.

Throughout these risk-taking activities we will occasionally be required to pivot to achieve the outcomes we desire. Our ability to pivot in the right direction comes from perseverance of deliberate practice. In each of the 4 Pillars, the more we can take micro risks, pivot when required and continue to persevere with these actions the better we will get, and the easier life will be.

Why? Because life becomes easy when we stop looking for it to be easy.

Activities

1. What deep desire have you been holding back from the world? How can you begin to live that desire in a small way each day?

2. List a micro risk for each of the 4 Pillars that you will perform this week that are a little outside your comfort zone.

3. Record your thoughts and associated mindset in your journal to those risks before, during and after completing them. Analyze how your body felt, emotions you were feeling and predominant thought patterns.

4. What are some strategies or plans you can have to assist you to pivot when challenged in taking your micro risk? What challenges can you foresee? And how can you strategize to prepare for them?

5. Are you a rewards-oriented person? What reward can you grant yourself once you have completed these challenges?

Week 4: Overcoming Setbacks

The greater the obstacle,
the more glory in
overcoming it.
– Moliere, French playwright

Failure and setback are consistent companions on the journey of self-development. The more we progress, the more the momentum builds, and the larger risks we undertake. The potential for failure also increases. At some point along the 4 Pillars journey, we reach a critical threshold that challenges us beyond anything we have encountered before.

Week Four is the halfway point in establishing new habits and often the most challenging. Our initial enthusiasm and willpower have diminished and by undertaking micro risks, we will have experienced setbacks in one or more of the Pillars. We might even begin questioning ourselves through negative self-talk or our fire of desire may have had water thrown on it from an outside source. Within these moments of greatest challenge, we must reconnect with our foundation to find a way to continue to push forward.

Moving Forward

As with most challenges we face, fear makes obstacles appear bigger than they are. Our imaginations focus on negative outcomes and build them into monsters that prevent us from taking action. We can convince ourselves we're better off playing it safe at the expense of our happiness and growth.

At some point in our journey in mastering the 4 Pillars, we will encounter a monumental setback with the potential to derail our best efforts. It will feel like the universe is punishing us and sabotaging our efforts. This may even happen time and time again. We might injure ourselves while exercising or get a medical diagnosis that scares us. An important relationship may end, or a financial loss will occur, prompting us to fall into despair.

THIS IS LIFE.

Setbacks and failure occur for everybody, every day. Our mind, as our greatest source of inspiration, can also be our greatest enemy. Negative thought patterns lead to negative feelings and behaviours. According to research undertaken by the National Science Foundation, we have anywhere between 12,000-60,000 thoughts per day with up to 80% of them negative. Surprisingly, 95% of those thoughts were repetitive thoughts from the day before. STOP. By the time we are 35 years old, 95% of our thoughts are repetitive. We are literally thinking the same thoughts day in and day out. Each day is a repetition of thoughts from the previous day. We may desire a healthy body, great relationships and financial freedom yet we are invariably sabotaging any efforts we make with outdated thoughts.

A similar study by Leahy (Cornell University, 2005) found that 85% of what we worry about never happens. Of those 15% of worries that did eventuate, 79% of subjects discovered they could handle the challenge better than they had expected, or that the challenge taught them a valuable lesson they appreciated. If we acknowledge that almost 97% of our worries are baseless and result from an unfounded negative mindset, we can imagine how our lives would change if we consciously attempted to replace negative thoughts with positive ones and focused more on the present instead of the future.

Cognitive Behaviour Therapy (CBT) is a form of psycho-social intervention that examines the relationship between our thoughts, feelings and behaviours. It has gained mainstream acceptance as an approach for tackling disorders such as anxiety and depression. With some knowledge of CBT, we can analyse our thoughts, feelings and behaviours when setbacks occur, and consciously devise a plan to get back on track.

Seth Gillihan, in *Retrain Your Brain: Cognitive Behavioural Therapy in 7 Weeks* (2017), identifies that when a setback occurs, negative thoughts flood our brain and impact our feelings and behaviours. These negative thoughts may not necessarily be based on any factual information and unless checked early, have the capacity to strengthen within us. So how do we overcome these negative thoughts? By growing awareness of our thought patterns, asking reflective questions and drawing our focus back to winning the moment.

Winning the Moment

Winning the moment is a positive self-talk strategy useful when we face challenging events. Winning each moment means doing our very best and feeling good in the present. It means relinquishing the 'What if …' thoughts of future outcomes and focusing the mind directly on what is occurring in front of us.

In committing our short-term plans, we cultivate the best version of ourselves in each moment. We choose to focus all our energy on being present in whatever task we are doing. In driving our car to conversing with a friend, concentrating on that moment suffocates negative thoughts and the fear that operates in what may or may not occur in the future.

Too often, we can get so far ahead of ourselves looking upon the long journey ahead, that we become paralyzed by inaction and fear. The short poem, "The Centipede's Dilemma" in Katherine Craster's *Pinafore Poems* (1871), resonates with this theme:

> A centipede was happy—quite!
> Until a toad in fun
> Said, "Pray, which leg moves after which?"

This raised her doubts to such a pitch,
She fell exhausted in the ditch
Not knowing how to run.

When the toad, in wonderment, asked the centipede how she managed to coordinate 100 legs to walk, the centipede realized she had never stopped to think about it. Accustomed to the freedom of moving along 100 legs simultaneously, the centipede was paralyzed with overthinking and collapsed.

This story reminds us that overthinking can impact our ability to make decisions in the present. The concept of paralysis by analysis was researched by psychologist, George Humphrey (1889-1966), who described the centipede syndrome as a psychological effect that occurs when we overthink. Instead of enjoying ourselves and following the path before us, we over-analyse the best options, resulting in no action at all. It's like standing at the crossroads of an important decision, thinking of all the options and getting run over by a bus!

Winning each moment means focusing on the next set or rep while working out in the gym or the next mile before us. It means doing what we can today to nourish our relationships without harbouring any long-term expectations on how we think everything should be. With finances, winning the moment could mean putting aside an extra $5 into our savings or not making that impulse purchase. Finally, winning the moment is about creating a consciously positive mindset and drawing our attention into the present without fearfully bracing for the future.

Developing Grit

Developing grit, resilience or the ability to bounce back when setbacks occur is a character trait we can all build. The foundations of grit are built on passion and persistence, as described by Angela Duckworth in her *New York Times* bestselling book, *Grit* (2018). According to Duckworth, society likes to gloss over passion and persistence in favor of natural talent; talent that is often the result of countless individual elements carefully drilled into a habit over years. Duckworth states that superlative performance (or mastery) is the result of sustained effort and that passion or enthusiasm enables that effort to be sustained. It's the determination to keep going after a setback that ensures success.

When setbacks occur, talent is tested. William James, a Harvard psychologist, asserted in 1907 that there is a difference between potential and actualization and that most people live far within their limits while only a few individuals learn to push beyond them.

A setback is seen as a 'set-back' for individuals determined to create lives on their terms. It does not define them or prevent them from taking action and risks. As we all experience setbacks across the 4 Pillars, our ability to summon and sustain our passion and internal fire of desire to keep taking action and moving forward is what counts. This a growth mindset. This is grit.

Ego

Setbacks impact our sense of self. The ego is the mind's representation of who we believe we are and how life should be. If our experience of life is different from our ego's viewpoint of how things 'should be' or we experience a setback, it can create inner conflict.

Have you ever tried to make a deal with the universe? Saying or thinking something along the lines of, 'If you give me this... I will do that'? As children, we made these deals and felt disappointed if we didn't get what we wanted. What if we imagined for a moment that the universe was ready and willing to give us exactly what we wanted, perhaps even more, yet our egos stood in the way of receiving it?

The strategies we implement to overcome setbacks—the rituals, habits and support—are not to force or bargain with the universe to yield to us. Instead, they clear our in-built resistance to allow great things to happen. We're cleaning away the dirt that has prevented our greatness from shining. Once we scrub away distortions and limitations contrived by our ego, we see ourselves more clearly. Our desires, our mastery of the 4 Pillars and everything else is already there—with setbacks as challengers to test how badly we desire success.

Weekly Reflection

What setback or challenge have you faced this week? How have those setbacks impacted your mindset and ability to move forward in creating a life on your terms?

Setbacks can potentially impact our ego, desire and mindset. Remember a setback is irrelevant; it's our choice in how we frame and respond to it that determines our success. When we respond consciously with compassion and action to setbacks, we develop grit. Winning each moment entails a consistent redirection of focus toward the present.

Our ego can separate us from the state of flow with distortions of reality and by seeding us with fear. In mastering each of the 4 Pillars, our ego may even sabotage our efforts if we are not considerate of its nature. When we stop and take a step back to reflect on our thoughts, we can determine who is in control of our ego and consequently direct it on a path of our choosing.

No one likes to fail, yet experiencing setbacks are an essential part of the 4 Pillars process and experiencing life itself. Regarding our bodies, working with setbacks builds stronger muscles. Learning to move beyond the comfort zone enables muscles to grow to meet increasing demand. Even our relationships require risks to facilitate growth. Investing in financial markets has obvious risks and there are no guarantees when we begin investing into ourselves.

We will fail many times throughout the 4 Pillars journey. In the attempt to improve ourselves and our life failure or setbacks will occur. Our challenge is to develop a mindset that embraces setbacks: a mindset not defined by any one external event, a mindset grounded in the belief that through our daily rituals and habits we have the inherent capacity to create a life we desire.

Overcoming Setbacks – A Personal Account: Covid-19

In March 2020, our world changed. COVID-19 swept the world at an alarming rate, forcing governments to implement strict lockdowns. Large cities became ghost towns overnight as all non-essential work, travel and gatherings were banned. People raided shops hoarding non-perishable items and displayed the very worst of human nature. Our world changed, and we were confronted with an unprecedented setback.

In Japanese literature, the word for crisis or danger also implies opportunity. In searching through every crisis and finding opportunities, our perspectives can shift to a higher plane. It takes a controlled mindset to see beyond the initial setback, but in these moments, success is guaranteed. It's not what happens to us that matters—what matters is how we respond.

Fear is physical, especially during uncertain times. If our body is functioning optimally, we reduce the effects fear has upon it. If there is peace within the body, there can be peace within the mind. Without peace, disease or a state of 'dis-ease' begins.

Under lockdown regulations, maintaining progress on the body pillar meant outdoor training and home body weight exercises such as push-ups, chin ups and squats. For me, four in the morning became the new alarm time which meant additional sleep and recovery. Rising early, going to sleep early and maintaining a disciplined approach to nutrition and hydration were my essential rituals to maintain when building a comeback.

With new social distancing laws, contact with other people and maintaining relationships was challenging under COVID restrictions. Zoom, email, phone and texts provided an outlet to support and check in with significant people in my life. Many of us reconnected with lost contacts and extended our care for others.

Personal relationships were under considerable stress. Family breakdown and domestic violence increased in a society without many positive coping mechanisms. Support and gentleness were required. Conversations grew deeper, as there was nowhere to go. Anxieties, insecurities and feelings were shared as debriefing and pressure release strategies. In times of challenge, our deep relationships support and nurture us as we also strive to support and nurture others.

The financial uncertainty brought by the lockdowns was the greatest setback for many. Overnight, dependable income stopped but expenses remained. Investments halved as economies shut and borders closed. Fear was real but also once-in-a-lifetime opportunities emerged. Maintaining a safety net of additional savings over the years provided a financial buffer for many, and a feeling of certainty. The share market had gone on sale and now was the time to capitalize. These financial decisions, in the time of great uncertainty, set the foundation for future financial success.

The mindset we are cultivating through the 4 Pillars sees opportunities and acts on them in times of setbacks. American investment guru Warren Buffet states, 'Be fearful when others are greedy and greedy when others are fearful.' We insulate ourselves from the negative, media invasion and focus on ourselves, our relationships and our immediate environment. We use our time to build our mindset in preparation for a comeback.

A setback does not define us, what does define us is our ability to respond positively when a setback occurs.

Activities

1. What setbacks have you encountered so far on the 4 Pillars journey? How have you responded to these setbacks both internally through your thoughts and externally through your actions? Record these in your journal.

2. Within the process of CBT, our thoughts, feelings and behaviours are linked together. List examples from your actions this week where you can see this cycle in action?

3. What strategies can you focus on to develop your own grit or resilience in the face of setbacks?

4. What are your strengths? List five of your strongest character traits that serve you when challenges arrive.

Week 5: Discipline Equals Freedom

Show me how you do one thing,
and I'll know how you do everything.
– Pedram Shojai, author & Taoist Abbot

Our imagination to create a better life begins with vision. A vision is shaped by the tasks we set and reshaped by the setbacks we overcome. It is further sharpened through the consistent performance of completing the seemingly unimportant tasks. These 1% activities are simple to do but often the easiest to forget. This is discipline. Completing these simple activities with energy and enthusiasm week in and week out. Being disciplined transforms our being. Through this transformation, we gain mastery over ourselves—the ultimate experience of freedom.

Becoming disciplined across the 4 Pillars is a skill to be embraced. Like any new skill it requires a foundation of knowledge and understanding to appreciate the common obstacles.

The Meaning of Discipline

The word discipline comes from the word 'disciple' which means to 'learn or to follow.' Through the art of 'learning and following,' we begin to set ourselves free. This is a significant understanding and something to reflect upon. In what areas of life can you become a disciple in following a higher path? Is it in creating a health body? Fulfilling relationships? Abundant finances? Or a firm mindset? Perhaps it's working towards creating the best version of yourself and living from a place of love and gratitude?

To become a disciplined person, we must first reject

laziness. Completing the activities, we know we should be doing even when we don't feel like doing them. There will be many times along the 4 Pillars journey when we don't feel like exercising, speaking kindly to others or saving our money. Our mind will come up with a myriad of excuses to justify why it is ok not to do something. Being disciplined is doing the activity regardless. By completing our daily rituals to the highest standard, we create freedom from negative thoughts and self-doubt. We consciously choose what to learn, how to spend our time and the people in our network and inner circle. Being disciplined is a choice and the choice is ours. Unless we have the focus to embrace a disciplined life, our desires will always remain as desires.

As we begin to show the results of our effort, people will comment on our discipline. It might be our improved health, relationships or expanding financial resources. Regardless of the areas, responding with gratitude and humility strengthens our character. It is uncommon to embrace a disciplined life, particularly across all 4 Pillars, yet as we have seen by now with small steps, performed with passion and consistency anything is possible.

If the word discipline carries negative connotations, replace it with another. Committed, dedicated and devoted also describe our ongoing actions. All these words signify inner resolve to continue moving forward. They also signify a decision to cut off distractions.

Write down and describe what these words mean for you and select the word that most fits your desired state. Call upon this imagery in times of challenge. When a work colleague offers birthday cake or there is a sale on large screen TVs, how would a person 100% committed to progress in health or finances respond?

Presence and Discipline

How does presence enhance discipline? Being present is not some mystical super-sensitive state. It is relaxing into what is occurring in front of our eyes and welcoming the moment. We can grow our awareness into presence in any moment. Right now, consider your posture, breath and what you have just been reading. To practice presence, try adjusting your posture, exhaling completely and then inhaling once again, drawing new breath, energy, and vitality into your being. This is presence. Presence is bringing this new energy and clarity to our body.

Often in conversations can we tell when others aren't present. We observe a lack of eye contact, signals from their body language such as checking the time, or an apparent lack of interest in what we are saying. We all have times when our minds move ahead of the present and discipline draws us back to the present.

The yogis have a Sanskrit term for mindful focus, *Viveka*, meaning discriminate discernment. It means consciously choosing where our focus lies in each moment. We train our minds to be aware of the choices presented before us and then make the best decision.

Conscious breathing is the most basic practice for growing presence, and we can start today. If the average person takes between 17,000-24,000 breaths per day, focusing on our breathing, particularly in times of stress, is an effective strategy.

Professional athletes use conscious breathing methods to bring themselves into the present moment and flow state. They write reminders on their wrists to create a trigger to anchor themselves back to the present moment.

What reminders or triggers can you use to help stay present throughout the course of the day?

Reminders can range from post-it notes on the bathroom

mirror to jewellery that inspires you with a message and brings awareness to your actions. Do an inventory of your workplace and home and see if there's a place where you can leave a few of these reminders. They are a powerful reminder of the life you are creating and a visual representation of your growing consciousness.

Discipline Equals Freedom

The term 'discipline equals freedom' was coined by author and retired Navy SEAL, Jocko Willink, in *Extreme Ownership* (2021). It appears contradictory, that being disciplined in completing our rituals equates a sense of freedom but being disciplined in our rituals is one method we can use to bring ourselves into the present.

Have you ever let your routines and rituals slip while on holidays or on vacation? During the first few days, you enjoy the extra time, space or energy but after the initial break, you may have felt restless and edgy. Perhaps negative self-talk and future thinking began to surface as well.

Socrates, one of the founders of Western philosophy is attributed with the saying, 'An undisciplined life is an insane life.'

Read that quote again.

Reflect on its wisdom and what it means to you.

In which areas of the 4 Pillars are you currently most undisciplined? Is it your body, your relationships, finances or mindset? List out several potential ways you see your discipline slip and pair them with some strategies to keep your focus this week.

Discipline and Patience

Discipline requires patience. Just as a young child makes many attempts in learning to walk, so must we in cultivating a life on our terms. Patience is a skillset that can be practiced through each of the 4 Pillars and applied to experiences that happen throughout our day. It begins with disciplining our mindset and is tested through failure. Patience is the capacity to accept or tolerate these failures without losing one's discipline.

The discipline required to develop patience comes from understanding our triggers. When our partner is running late for our dinner date, or our investments appear stagnated it is easy to become annoyed and lose our patience and discipline. Our amygdala fires, resulting in unconscious or fear-based decisions. We lash out at our partner or make a reckless decision with our money. Patience is the ability to see through the fog and continue regardless.

The *Chinese Bamboo Tree* story is an example of discipline and patience in action.

> To flourish, The Chinese Bamboo Tree requires daily nurturing; water, sunshine, fertile soil and an optimal growing environment. In the first year, there are no visible signs of growth. In the second year, again, no signs of activity or development. And the third and fourth, still no signs above the soil. Discipline is required in attending to the tree and patience is tested.
>
> Finally in the fifth year – magic! There is growth…and what growth it is! The Chinese Bamboo Tree grows 60-80 feet (20-30m) in just six weeks!

The question is: Does the Chinese Bamboo Tree grow 80 feet in six weeks or 5 years?

The answer of course is 5 years. During that time, it was developing its root system and a stable foundation for future growth. Had the farmer not the discipline to water and fertilize the tree during this time, even for a short period, it would have died.

This example is further demonstrated in society when a

new sensation makes a 'breakthrough' on the sporting field, experiences musical success with a number one hit or suddenly becomes the CEO of a large organization. The media will portray this 'come from nowhere' scenario as an overnight discovery. They will gloss over the years of preparation the individual has put into themselves to be in a position for this success. The countless hours of practice, rehearsals and study forms the character that allows these opportunities to present themselves. Discipline is the continual work to prepare and to be ready for these opportunities. Jeff Bezos sums up success nicely, 'All overnight success takes about 10 years.'

Discipline within the 4 Pillars requires patience. Patience with our health, patience in growing our relationships, patience with our developing finances and finally patience with our mindset. We require a strong foundation of discipline to sustain success. The length of time to experience the success we desire is irrelevant, it's the discipline in maintaining consistency with our rituals that is the lesson. Without the discipline in maintaining consistency, we will never achieve our desires. We will never know how close we might be to that big breakthrough if we give up.

We Get What We Focus On

Many lessons occur each day if we only take the time to tune into their messages. An incident may happen on our way to work or an exchange of words with a colleague may leave us feeling unsettled. We might directly observe the destruction of our environment or a negative turn in the economy. All these incidents impact our mindset leaving negative impressions.

Repeatedly, we are conditioned to place our attention on negative outcomes.

In changing our focus from these negatives, we discipline our minds to see the deeper lessons and positive messages that are available to us. We switch off the television and are selective in the media we consume. We discipline our mind to avoid these distractions from the path we are choosing to take. Why? Because focus equals power.

If you have had a challenging day this week, at the end of the day write out the negatives and deliberately write out the positives. For example, 'I have come to see that my manager is a narcissist (negative)…means that I am learning (positive) how to handle difficult personalities. I am now deliberately looking for a job where I am valued for my contribution to the workplace.' Another example is 'I made some unhealthy food choices throughout the day impacting my energy and vitality. I now recognize the impact such food has on my vitality and will ensure I have healthy food options available when I may require them.'

Weekly Reflection

Reflecting upon each day and week helps us examine our thoughts, behaviours and the results we are experiencing. If the results are not in alignment with our goals, we can change our point of focus. Choosing to focus on the positive lessons we are learning, the growth we are experiencing and the progress we are making, conditions the mind to experience the beauty and preciousness that is around us.

The word discipline is not about sacrificing joy and happiness for relentless effort and grind. It is about creating a mindset that is firm, steady and focused on living our desires and consistently taking small actions towards living them. With the right understanding, we can embrace a disciplined life and mindset, resulting in freedom of thinking and fulfilment of desires.

Activities

1. Where is your focus throughout the day? Future, past or present? Write about the moments when you slipped into the past or raced into the future. What was it like for you? Did you see a negative pattern in your thoughts or was it positive? Explore.

2. Write down in your journal what each of these words mean for you. Which best describes the actions you are taking and your desire for success?

- Disciplined
- Committed
- Dedicated
- Devoted

3. What activities help bring you into the present moment?

4. What areas within the 4 Pillars where you are currently living an undisciplined or even an 'insane' life?

5. Do you believe that you can create a life on your terms? What beliefs prevent you from living this way?

6. Where can you begin to embrace a disciplined life to set yourself free? What does that look like for you? Write about a time when you experienced discipline that gave you more freedom.

Week 6: Developing Faith

> Faith is taking the first step,
> even when you don't see the whole staircase.
> – Dr. Martin Luther King, Baptist Minister & activist

'Time stands still for no one,' reminds us to be continually on the move with all 4 Pillars. There are only ever two states of being: moving toward our goals or away from them.

As we enter Week Six, we may get a little too comfortable in performing our rituals and habits. We might look for short cuts, our focus is elsewhere and our risk-taking activities have subsided. It can also mean we've settled into a fixed rather than strived to maintain a growth mindset. We may even be slipping back into old patterns of behaviour and thinking.

This week, we draw on our faith. Developing and nurturing a sense of faith in ourselves and in something larger than us enables us to overcome each setback we encounter, maintain our sense of discipline and continue to take action. Faith is believing without seeing and an individual with faith is unstoppable.

Faith

Faith is easy when life is progressing for us, but what happens when we don't see results or, worse yet, we stumble and feel we are regressing? What is faith and how do we develop unshakeable faith? Is there even a place for faith in our contemporary world?

At this point in the 4 Pillars journey, we are refining our rituals and disciplining our actions. We find balance and harmony in our pursuit of creating a life on our terms. Yet, there might still be a missing link, an energy that propels us forward in taking the strategic actions and risks. Faith is that link. Faith compels us to transcend what we see. It allows us to believe our actions will come to fruition.

Faith is the basis for many of the world's spiritual traditions. *Sraddha* is the Indian Sanskrit word for faith and means clarity of mind and belief in the goal. In the New Testament, Corinthians 5:7 states, 'For we live by faith, not by sight,' and, in the Old Testament, Hebrews 11:1 reads, 'Now faith is the assurance of things hoped for, the conviction of things not seen.'

John Bishop in his article 'Faith', published in the *Stanford Encyclopedia of Philosophy*, (1995) explored the aspects of faith into three broad categories: affective, cognitive and practical. The affective component of faith includes a state of confidence and trust. It's an internal attitude towards an external belief. When we feel confident in our ability to achieve a set outcome, our internal values, beliefs and mindset align with what we are attempting to achieve. In simple terms, our head, heart and spirit are aligned with certainty.

The cognitive component of faith reflects the knowledge that what we are setting out to achieve has been done before. If we observe other people who create a life on their terms, then it is more possible for us to create ours as well. We listen to their stories, see their material successes and have the confidence that we can create the lives we choose also.

What happens then, if what we are setting out to achieve has never been done before, such as the trailblazers, inventors and athletes who expand human potential? One example is Roger Bannister, who broke the record for the four-minute mile. Until 1954, it was widely believed that no human could possibly run that fast. Athletes, physicians and the public all thought it was foolish to attempt what they believed was impossible. Since Bannister broke the four-minute mile record, thousands of athletes, including high school students, have also broken it. Once people intellectually understood it was possible, it created the faith that they could do it as well.

Roger Bannister incorporated visualization techniques, imagining himself breaking the record and running a mile under four minutes. By repeatedly imagining himself breaking the record, he created certainty within his body and mind. He effectively developed his affective component of faith to such an extent that it was enough to overcome any intellectual doubt he may have had.

The final element of faith demands a practical response from us. Faith requires accompanied action. The more positive action we take, the more our faith grows. Practical faith is built from action and small, Kaizen steps are the best starting point.

Reflect on your current level of faith in creating a life on your terms. Do you believe it is possible to create a life on your terms and if so, how is it represented in your daily rituals? Do you listen to and read stories from people who have achieved remarkable results and feel inspired that you can achieve success as well? Do you visualize the life you desire and take daily action in bringing those visions to reality?

Faith through Action

If we find ourselves growing too comfortable and stagnating, seek advice from friends and colleagues to support our sense of motivation. Our network of friends can offer suggestions that we may have overlooked, and we can also look to create a new path.

Alex Banayan, in *The Third Door* (2018), presents the concept of creating new actions and opportunities by finding the third door. Banayan uses the analogy of a nightclub with three entrances accessible for people to achieve their desires. Most people line up and wait, hoping to get in. A small percentage are VIPs slip through without lining up. Then he cites the third door—for those prepared to jump out of line, run around the back, bang on the door, crack open a window or sneak through the kitchen. This door, like life, are for those who are continually prepared to take risks and have the faith that they will somehow make it through. This door requires courage.

Most people are stuck, waiting for the right conditions before they act. They line up patiently, hoping for that magical signal when resistance falls away. This will never happen. We must be the ones who create the conditions for a better life through our continual actions.

What conditions are you waiting for that are holding you back from living your best life now? Do they involve health, relationships, finances, mindset or a combination of all four? How can you move beyond these limitations and begin living from these desired states? What actions can you take today?

The third door encourages us to look at our challenges with new eyes. To see a different perspective and opportunity that may currently be disguised as a problem. We use our conditioned mindset to broaden our focus and scan for alternative actions. Asking ourselves open ended questions and providing space for the mind to answer is an approach that often yields results. Questions such as 'What is my deepest desire? or how can I 10X my income this year?' are questions we can continually ask ourselves. By asking these questions, we are deliberately challenging our mind. And our mind loves a challenge. These questions need time and space for a response. You may be surprised by what comes up if you listen attentively.

Luck

While luck is associated with good fortune, it can also be associated with a healthy body, great relationships, strong finances and a positive mindset. But is luck real? Are some people born luckier than others? Or is it an excuse by those who aren't achieving their potential?

Good fortune favours those who create supportive conditions within their internal mindsets; those who condition their minds to see opportunities like the 'third door.' In other words, we create luck with a controlled mindset. Within every new experience, we shape our response through the language we use. The following Chinese story explores good and bad luck and how it is truly determined by perspective.

> Once there was a farmer who used an old horse to till his fields until the horse escaped into the hills. When the farmer's neighbours discovered his loss, they sympathized with the old man over his bad luck.
>
> The farmer replied, 'Bad luck? Good luck? Who knows?'
>
> A week later, the horse returned with a herd of horses from the hills and this time the neighbours congratulated the farmer on his good luck.
>
> His reply was, 'Good luck? Bad luck? Who knows?'
>
> Then, when the farmer's son was attempting to tame one of the wild horses, he fell off its back and broke his leg. Everyone thought this was very bad luck.
>
> The farmer again replied, 'Bad luck? Good luck? Who knows?'
>
> Some weeks later, the army marched into the village and conscripted every able-bodied youth they found there. When they saw the farmer's son with his broken leg, they let him off.

Was that good luck or bad luck? Who knows?

All our experiences have the potential to be labeled bad luck or good luck. Sometimes a bad experience may be a good one in disguise.

Would you consider yourself 'lucky or unlucky' in each of the 4 Pillars? Reflect and record the factors or events that have led to this way of thinking. Record previous habits or thoughts that have also contributed to this way of thinking.

For example, you may record that you felt unlucky inheriting genetics that make losing weight more challenging than for others. Next, shift the thinking to record the gift or 'luck' that you have been granted in accepting this challenge. Thoughts would include enhanced compassion for others who also feel challenged, a determination to be an example for your family or the gift of understanding the importance of health and wellbeing. Undertake this task for each of the 4 Pillars and reflect upon any areas where you have felt unlucky or disadvantaged.

Through this activity, we can identify thought patterns that have been holding us back. We might be labeling events as unlucky when, with a shift in mindset, we see the gift that has presented itself to us.

New insights and actions come to us when we change our perspective.

Perspective

Perspective is our view of the world and the lens by which we view it from. Two individuals can share the same experience, yet their perspective of that experience might be completely different. During the 19th century, Alfred Adler developed the field known as Alderian Psychology. Along with Freud and Jung, Adler was one of the three giants of psychology at the time.

Alderian Psychology is a realisation that the meaning we associate with events will determine our sense of self. The event itself is irrelevant, our interpretation of that event will shape our identity and behaviour. It implies that our perspective of any event is open to interpretation. To live with this mindset takes great courage.

Perspective brings liberation. We are not bound by our past and are free to shape events however we choose them to be. Some may say that this is living in a fairy world and not facing up to the reality of life. Yet aren't we already living this way? We constantly take our past experiences and overlay them with anything remotely similar, expecting the same response. We anticipate the rejection or sore body before the event and believe that is the way the world works. Alderian Psychology accepts the events that occur and selects a response that creates harmony, peace and happiness within the body and mind.

Try this activity the next time someone beeps at you while driving. Pretend, or take the perspective, that the person beeping at you is not annoyed by your actions—in fact, they are a friend that you haven't seen for years and are desperately trying to get your attention. How does this change of perspective impact your body, emotions, and mind? Are you a little calmer, happier and perhaps even excited? This change of perspective will automatically illicit a different response from you all because you made the decision to view an event differently.

These types of actions require conditioning of our mindset and taking a step back from events before responding. How would your health, relationships and finances change if you took a moment to consciously look at events from a different perspective?

Weekly Reflection

In mastering the 4 Pillars, sometimes it can be difficult to quantify our progress. We may feel like we are not making progress at all. Faith asserts that we continue to act when there is no external progress to be seen. It also takes courage to trust ourselves, trust our skills and resilience, and believe that everything will unfold in the direction in which we strive.

At times we may have to look for the third door to catch some momentum again. Feeling stuck or stale in our health, relationships, finances and mindset is an indicator that we have grown comfortable and different actions are required.

Luck is a word used for people who do not appreciate the interrelatedness of life. Events occur for and against us that appear to have no logical meaning. When we refuse to label events by grounding ourselves back into our rituals, we maintain our confidence and determination. From this controlled mindset, a change of perspective results in new insights that inspire new actions.

Activities

1. How strongly do you believe in your goals and your ability to create a life on your terms? Are you 100% committed, disciplined in your actions and developing your faith? Is there any belief preventing you from feeling and acting with this certainty? Plan time this week to reflect in your journal your commitment to creating a life on your terms.

2. Have you experienced a lag or a sense of stagnation this week? Are you still taking risks across the 4 Pillars? List a few that you have not yet taken that you would like to take this week and next.

3. What actions or rituals can you create to develop your faith? Can you use your imagination more or incorporate visualization?

4. Where can you find your own 'third door' for each of the 4 Pillars to overcome present obstacles?

5. What are your thoughts around luck? Do you believe you were born lucky/unlucky and that you have the power to create your own luck?

6. How often do you follow your intuition? Can you tune into this awareness more when making decisions?

7. What areas of life require a change of perspective? A perspective that will encourage peace, harmony and happiness within?

Week 7: Celebrating Now & Resetting

Life should not only be lived,
it should be celebrated.
– Osho, Indian mystic

Let's assess how your life has changed over the last six weeks.

In some ways, you are a different person from the one who began this program six weeks ago. Your environment has changed through the never-ending changing of the seasons along with trillions of cells in your body. Daily experiences have reshaped your thinking along with additional knowledge and experience you have acquired. You are constantly changing and evolving in unique and special ways. This week, we assess how we have changed, the positive and not so positive aspects of change and acknowledge the challenges we have overcome in celebrating our life now.

Celebrating Now

What are you doing to celebrate your life right now?

Have you been dancing, spending time with friends and loved ones or sitting quietly in nature? Have you had a massage or a haircut? Have you found time to walk mindfully on grass during your lunch break or stare up in amazement at the stars?

How have you rewarded yourself for the progress you've made so far?

How have you been kind to yourself?

Doing something we love is a great way to celebrate life. Providing occasions for ourselves also gives us energy for our next challenge. Each day, there are countless opportunities to embrace and celebrate life. When we place our focus on our celebration of life, life becomes a celebration.

For achievers and those focused on creating a life on their terms, taking time out to find some joy can be challenging. For many of us, we somehow feel better about ourselves when we are fully engaged in the 'battle' of life. Slaying conflict and forcing ourselves to overcome each hurdle thrown at us keeps us motivated and determined, but this is physically, emotionally and mentally draining work. In this never-ending battle, we might even be avoiding the very best time of our lives: the present.

Celebrating life creates space for reflection on our achievements and acknowledge the effort we make in improving ourselves, particularly when moving from one life event to another. We end one chapter of life, celebrate and savor it before moving onto the next. We end one day, celebrate and savor it with gratitude before moving onto the next to celebrate our lives now.

The first activity for this week is to dedicate some time for celebration. Take a morning off from rituals and do an activity that you haven't done for some time. Play in the park with the kids, read the newspaper or reset in nature.

Contemplating Death

Contemplating our inevitable death can be the catalyst for a new course in living. We are all going to die. It is something that unities us all. Yet few people use this one certainty of life as a catalyst for living now.

It's ironic that in a chapter where we aim to celebrate the life we have now, we reflect on our death. Yet that is exactly the task that can inspire us to appreciate what we have now and not to delay our happiness for an imaginary future. The notion that we have time prevents us from acting and appreciating what we have now.

If you knew the moment your death would occur, what

impact would that knowledge have on your living now? If you had a day, a week, a month, or a year left to live, what would change? Would you worry over the activities that currently occupy most of your thoughts and feel anxious of missed opportunities and suppressed desires?

Or perhaps you were confined to a hospital bed and couldn't go out to see the sky? To feel the sunlight on your body, to watch the stars at night or smell the coming rain? These are everyday events happening now that one day we will not be here to appreciate.

Many of our daily fears and troubles melt in the face of death. We cannot change our past and our future is yet to be written but we can do something about living with discipline and faith now. Life is not a rehearsal so why not embrace our best living?

The death reflection is an opportunity to contemplate the transitory nature of life and the impermanence of everything. Our body, our relationships and all our wealth will pass. Life is not something you get; it's something you experience. Therefore, we create a life of worth now, embrace the discipline of that process and experience life while we can.

There is a story of a great yogi who said that every moment of his life he felt as though a sword were suspended above his head by a spiderweb. He lived his life with the awareness that he was that close to death.

Death can be the greatest teacher. It is not morbid thinking about death. The morbidity comes from living the same life, year after year waiting for some magical time when everything falls into place. There is no perfect timing. We must create the perfect timing and act before our time runs out. We can let our impending death serve as inspiration for celebrating and enjoying our life.

Contemplating death is an activity to appreciate the impermanence of life and assist us in living more fully. It can provide perspective for our life and challenge us to absorb the experience of being alive. Contemplating death can be a catalyst to reach out to those we love and tell them how much we love and appreciate them.

Resetting

We all need a break, a moment to withdraw and reset. We can reset by spending time in nature. Research from nature. com indicates that spending 120 minutes a week in nature is associated with improved mental and physical wellbeing. Whether through one long or several shorter intervals, the positive benefits of time in nature are reductions in stress, obesity and cardiovascular disease along with better wellbeing and improved cognitive development for children. Time in nature isn't just a break and a reward, it's also beneficial.

Negative ions are abundant in nature and neutralize many of the effects of the contaminated environment we live in. Potentially detrimental aspects of electromagnetic fields in buildings and homes (due to internal wiring) and carrying our smart or electronic devices with us all the time can create weakness in the body. Time in nature provides an opportunity for negative ions to cleanse these positive ions, purifying the blood and cell membranes. Spending time in nature is a simple, effective strategy to reset after a challenging day.

Physical activity is another useful strategy for resetting the body and mind. Intense physical activity floods our body and mind with positive endorphins, reducing our perception of pain and increasing our positive emotions. No matter how challenging a day, going for a run will always help us feel better about ourselves.

There will be moments throughout our day when doing physical activity may not be possible. During these times, when our mindset is triggered and we feel ourselves spiraling into negative thought patterns, a few moments by ourselves can provide space to regather ourselves, focus our attention on winning the moment and to practice deep breathing. We can go to the bathroom or head outside where we can have a few uninterrupted moments to practice positive self-talk and gratitude.

For the second activity this week, trial reset strategies and their effectiveness in shifting negative thoughts and energy. The activities listed above are a good starting point but also consider laughter, listening to music or any other creative outlet. Creative pursuits allow us to express ourselves more fully, increasing feel good hormones and endorphins. Photography, painting, writing, building and construction projects are other examples of creative outlets.

Our only limitations are the limitations that exists in our mind.

Feeling Good for Success

If you had to rate it, how good do you feel today? And yesterday? Assess your average 'feel good' state for this week.

A practical goal in working towards mastery of the 4 Pillars is practicing the ability to feel good for no specific reason. Feeling good means that we are energized by what we are doing, at peace in our surroundings and involved in meaningful pursuits. We find enjoyment in the company of others as well as peace and contentment by ourselves.

We may already know people in our life who walk into a room and radiate magnetic energy and success. No problem or issue is too big for those who seem to float above the congestion of everyday life. They have conditioned themselves to be in peak state and feeling good is natural for them.

For this week, imagine that any challenges you face are opportunities to practice feeling outstanding regardless of the environment. Remind yourself that these challenges are gifts in disguise. Throughout the day, ask yourself these questions:

- Does this feel good to me?
- Why does this feel good/bad?
- Can I feel good regardless of what events are happening around me?

Nothing great can happen from a state of fear, frustration or depression.

Feeling good and celebrating the now are reflections we all need to remember. In pursuit of our desires, these states provide life and energy required to overcome the obstacles we face and take us to new levels of being. Just as our habits and rituals provide the framework for success, cultivating our ability to find joy in what are doing enriches our day. A mindset directed towards feeling good is a mindset that is clear, focused and energized when challenges arise.

Weekly Reflection

From the moment we leave our home in the morning, until our return in the evening, we are changing and along the journey of the 4 Pillars, this change is conscious and deliberate. At this stage, we're embracing change and seeing ourselves grow. That's something to celebrate.

In mastering the 4 Pillars and creating a life on our terms we must continually realign our mindset and implement strategies to enable us to stay in our best state. Contemplating our inevitable death is one strategy that can assist us gain greater perspective on life. Celebrating what we do have in this moment rather than focusing on what we don't shifts our attention towards gratitude and cultivates a sense of joy. Resetting provides us with space and assists us in acknowledging our challenges alongside our gifts and our progress.

Feeling good for success makes a great motto. Feeling good for no reason creates new opportunities and allows fresh insights to come to us. When we celebrate the now, we are opening ourselves up to be in the best state possible, conditioning ourselves to remain positive, enthusiastic and energetic regardless of the environment.

Activities

1. How do you celebrate life? These can be small or grander gestures. What strategies can you implement to enrich your life with enjoyment each day?

2. What can you do to find the magic moments in the present moment?

3. Contemplate your impending death. What bold actions would you take if you had one week left to live?

4. Call, write or visit someone you haven't spoken to for a while and tell them you love them.

5. Try several different reset strategies throughout the week and describe the impact they have on your energy and mindset.

6. Spend time in nature this week.

7. Determine one activity you can do this week that you haven't done for a while that will make you feel good. An activity that was once your 'passion'. Reflect on your feelings whilst doing this activity. Can you make room to rekindle this passion?

Week 8: Living Your Best Life

Who you become tomorrow,
will be defined by what you do today.
– John Maxwell, speaker & author

Week Eight is the culmination of seven weeks of effort investing time and energy into your health, relationships, finances and mindset. By now, with continued persistence and action, results are evident. For some of us, these results might be difficult to quantify for others in our circle of friends and family, but they are clear for us. Only we truly know the changes that have occurred and the progress achieved over the last seven weeks.

Week Eight is the ending of one cycle of change and preparation for another. We appreciate that life is cyclical. As night follows day and the seasons change from summer to autumn, there is a never-ending cycle of growth, shedding and rebirth unfolding.

Throughout the last seven weeks you have changed. How you have changed depends upon the rituals you created, the intensity of the routines and risks, and the level of consistency in completing your plans. How you have changed depends on the challenges you faced and the enthusiasm and strategies you applied in overcoming them.

In life we don't get what we want; we get what we become. By investing in the 4 Pillars throughout the last eight weeks you have initiated the process of creating a life on your terms.

The Art of Fulfilment

Let's reflect upon the last seven weeks from a few angles.
Did you achieve the goals you set yourself seven weeks

ago? Were they too ambitious or too easy? Were the challenges overcome with enthusiasm, resilience and energy?

In short, can you measure continual progress in each of the 4 Pillars?

The science of achievement dictates that there are universal strategies we can all implement to improve our lives. Strategies such as eating nutritious food, appreciating the work of others we love and saving more than we spend all produce observable results. Universal in their application, these and many more strategies create success in our health, relationships, finances and mindset.

Just as we know certain strategies work, it does not mean they will work specifically for us or that we will be consistent in their application. When motivational speaker, Tony Robbins discusses the art of fulfilment, he indicates that selecting the right strategy is unique to every person and every objective. He also acknowledges that simply understanding the strategies of achievement alone will not bring success and happiness. Robbins emphasises the art of fulfilment or the ability to create the right psychology, or mindset, within us equates to 80% of the success formula. Even with the right strategy at our disposal, our mindset can either hold us back or propel us forward. In facing any challenge, it's our interpretation of events that determine how we respond.

Now is a good time to remember that success or failure in any one goal or event does not define who we are becoming. There is a much bigger picture at play. We may have struggled to complete some or all the activities we assigned ourselves. Or we may have smashed through our objectives and may be riding high on momentum. The 4 Pillars are about the long-haul, the lifelong journey, with all its ebbs and flows, and the culmination of our choices, actions and outcomes is the picture that defines us. The art of fulfillment teaches us that success comes from our small wins and our attitude towards improving ourselves and the lives of those we love.

Be More

Imagine for a moment that you are already a master of the 4 Pillars and have consciously created a life on your terms. How would you look, speak and act? More importantly, how would you feel? This internal state is the one we are approaching and practicing. We cannot wait for the external world to change before we do.

Our work over the last seven weeks entailed rituals and habits to assist us in changing ourselves for the better. We are determined to become the person we want to be now. We are driven to live each day with the energy and enthusiasm of a person who is already a master of the 4 Pillars.

In choosing to behave with the certainty of creating great health, fantastic relationships, an abundance of wealth and a strong and positive mindset, the path ahead grows clearer. If we already have great health, making conscious decisions around nutrition is easy. If we have fantastic and loving relationships, we will show gestures of love and not be offended if it is not reciprocated. If we have an abundance of wealth, we are open to sharing our abundance with others. If our mindset is strong, we demonstrate a growth mindset and are resilient when encountering challenges.

The culminating activity for Week Eight is to envision a day five years from now. Select a day five years from now and describe in minute detail each event that occurs throughout the day. Begin by waking in up bed. What type of bed is it? What is the color of the bed sheets? What are you wearing and are you alone or with someone? Be as specific as possible and write from a place of no limits. Proceed throughout your day and describe the activities you do, who you are doing them with and where you are doing them. Take time to complete this task. There is no rush. Remember, the more detailed you are the greater the clarity you hold. This is a fun activity, so let the imagination run wild.

The significance of this activity cannot be ignored. Your ability to create a life on your terms begins with an imagination of what your life can be. By visualizing this real day in the future, you are setting a course towards this new life.

Life reflects who we are internally. 'Being more' is not 'doing more,' where we exhaust ourselves physically and mentally each day with endless activities. 'Being more' is living our perfect life now with the assurance that life will provide inspiration and opportunity at the perfect time. Imagining a time in the future sets in place a motion from our consciousness of what is possible. With supportive rituals and developing belief, we are sharpening an internal focus that keeps us calm and consistent on our path to success.

Internal Focus, External Results

In a world of continuous distraction, our internal environment shapes our external reality. Our thoughts, feelings and beliefs generate our results because they determine our actions. If we are constantly thinking and feeling thoughts of fear and scarcity, our actions and results will reflect our anxiety. If we are constantly thinking, feeling and believing at our deepest level that we are the master of our life, our actions will naturally reflect it.

The activities from the last seven weeks have helped shaped our internal environment. Working from the outside to the inside. We created external rituals for our health, relationships and finances to support our internal mindset. We gained a deeper awareness of our mindset through these rituals and our awareness of this internal dialogue has grown.

By now, we know that saying no to external distractions requires courage with the endless competition vying for our attention. Media, work, family, friends, the list is endless. We've also learned that our inner game determines external success. Those who believe they can, will. Saying no is the courage to select the activities and rituals that draw us closer to being the person we desire. Saying no is powerful.

Week Eight invites space into our lives through saying no.

Where in your life right now do you need to say no? Do you need to say no to invitations, external distractions or any of the never-ending requests placed on your time?

It takes courage to say no. To risk judging ourselves and experience the rejection of others. Ichiro Kishimi and Fumitake Koga, in *The Courage to be Disliked* (2017), draw on Adlerian principles to confer that many of our problems stem from interpersonal relationships and our inability to say no. It's this inability to say no to external expectations from others, or our own intrusion into other people's lives that creates conflict. From health, relationship and financial choices, conflict exists when others intrude in our decisions, or we intrude in theirs. Freedom then, is to risk being disliked.

Saying no creates space and challenges many of our relationships. In responding to the little requests of our time, we say, 'Thank you and no I cannot do that.' We are not compelled to give reasons if we don't want to as this opens opportunities for others to bargain with us.

Creating space to say no is powerful. It takes great courage to say no.

Grace

The final contemplation on this 4 Pillars journey is the nature of grace. Grace transcends the mundane into magic. Along with faith, it's the invisible energy that vibrates through every one of us destined to live a magical life. Grace is appreciating that there are other, more powerful forces at play. It is acknowledging that we are part of a universal collective energy moving towards something that we cannot comprehend.

We cannot achieve everything we desire through sheer force alone. There comes a place where we can do everything humanly possible to shift changes in our direction, but grace allows that change to unfold. Grace allows us to accept that everything is happening for a reason. While we can have clearly defined goals and strategies, grace determines the ultimate outcome. Through practicing our daily actions and rituals with intent, we provide the opportunity for grace to touch our lives in a positive manner. The resilience we develop in responding to challenges with enthusiasm and determination also clears a pathway for grace to enter our lives.

In *The Alchemist* (1988) by Paul Coelho, the word grace is referred to as *maktub*, meaning 'it is written' in Arabic, and indicates that fate binds us to certain pathways. Some may call this destiny and become despondent of change. Why go to the effort of investing time, energy and resources into change when life is predestined?

With an appreciation of *maktub*, we can gracefully embrace change with trust and a solid foundation. We have the capacity to determine how we interpret life's events and move along its pathways. Every activity undertaken has the potential to be transformed into a mindful ritual. From brushing our teeth to driving our car, deliberate awareness brings the quality of grace to each moment.

Grace is liberation. Grace frees us from our disappointment and expectation that everything should go our way all the time. Grace fills us with wonder at the synchronicities and beauty of life.

Weekly Reflection

Our internal mindset always determines our external results. Win the inner game and external results flow. Week Eight in our cycle of change is a reflection on our progress and learning to say no to the never-ending distractions that can impede our progress. It is imagining a time in the not-too-distant future where we live the perfect existence. We are invited to reflect upon our internal and external progress over the past two months and take action to create more space within our lives.

Are you a better, richer, fuller and more resilient person now than you were eight weeks ago?

Can you appreciate the progress within your journey is both an internal and external game?

As we cultivate a deeper understanding of the strategies of success that work for us, we are growing to appreciate the art of fulfillment. The art that creates the internal environment that sees us continue to take bold actions. We know that doing more does not equate to being more and learning to say no to distractions helps us stay focused on the task of creating a life on our terms.

Grace allows us to appreciate that life is moving towards a higher destination outside of our awareness and control. Our efforts of self-development within the 4 Pillars grows more graceful as we perform rituals with greater awareness and intent.

Creating and embedding new rituals into habits takes time. It is a continual process of experimentation, action and reflection; a never-ending cycle and constant change.

Activities

1. How have you changed over the last seven weeks across the 4 Pillars? Use your journal to identify and write about the positive changes that you observe.

2. How have you struggled over the last seven weeks? Outline some ways to adapt your plans and pivot your approach to help you meet your goals.

3. In what areas of your life can you begin to say no? What does that look like and how will you communicate your boundaries to others in an assertive and authentic way?

4. If you say no to someone, what is your strategy if you feel you are being pushed or pressured in response? Remember that while it's exciting and inspiring to share details of your journey, you do not have to defend your decision to enrich your life. Some of your decisions will be met with resistance so have a plan to navigate that possibility and still stick to your original plan.

5. Can you visualise a day five years from now where you are living a beautiful experience on your terms? What does it look like?

6. Where has grace impacted your life over the last seven weeks? Have there been moments where you have encountered a new experience? When have you felt especially inspired? Write about those moments and explore the details that surround them.

Final Thoughts

Time.

From the first breath we take on this planet to our very last, the clock is ticking.

How we spend our time between these events determines the deepest quality of our lives. The actions we take, or fail to take, on a daily, weekly and monthly basis accumulate across the years and shape our lives.

How many days we have on this planet is unknown, but we can consciously influence their quality. Over the last eight weeks, the challenge has been laid for you to consciously create your life on your terms and live to your fullest potential. How you continue to learn, reflect and grow from this point forward determines the quality of your future.

The journey of the 4 Pillars offers an opportunity to take control of the main areas in our lives that have the greatest impact on our peace, happiness and success. A healthy body, happy relationships, sufficient finances and a strong and positive mindset affect our wellbeing entirely. We can obtain success in these areas with consistent, dedicated and enthusiastic approaches to improvement and flexibility in our practice. Our practice begins each day with our first thoughts in the morning and where they are directed. It continues throughout the day with our rituals and small actions and concludes with our final reflections as we fall asleep.

Creating a great body or lots of money will not make us happy. Creating rituals that lead to continual progress along the 4 Pillars will. Developing a positive mindset requires daily attention, and like a muscle, it must be consistently trained to attain results. The cumulative effect of this work brings us peace and harmony on the inside that draws peace and happiness to us from the outside.

In continually investing in yourself, you will discover that mastery of the 4 Pillars is possible. To master one's health, relationships, finances and mindset requires you to rise above common patterns and traps and to become an uncommon person: a person dedicated to living a life of their highest potential.

Further Readings

PART I

Chapter 1

Forbes, R. M., Cooper, A. R., & Mitchell, H. H. (1953). The Composition of the Adult Human Body as Determined by Chemical Analysis. *Journal of Biological Chemistry*, 203, 359-366.

Villoldo, A. (2019). *Grow a New Body: How Spirit and Power Plant Nutrients Can Transform Your Health*. California. Hay House.

Chapter 2

Buettner, D., & Skemp, S. (2016). Blue zones: lessons from the world's longest lived. *American Journal of Lifestyle Medicine* 10(5), 318-321.

Holloway, R. L. (1981). "Culture, Symbols, and Human Brain Evolution: A Synthesis." *Dialectical Anthropology* 5(4), 287-303.

Altman, I., & Taylor, D. A. (1973). *Social Penetration: The Development of Interpersonal Relationships*. Holt, Rinehart & Winston.

Morton, J. (2021). *Soldier: Respect is Earned*. London. Harper Collins Publishers.

Pomerantz, E. M., & Thompson, R. A. (2008). "Parents' Role in Children's Personality Development: The Psychological Resource Principle."

Chapter 3

Classon, G. S. (2020). *The Richest Man in Babylon*. New York. Sristhi Publishers & Distributors.

Fisher, M. (1991). *The Instant Millionaire: A Tale of Wisdom and Wealth*. California. New World Library.

Stanley, T. J. (1996). *The Millionaire Next Door: The Surprising Secrets of America's Wealthy*. Lanham. Taylor Trade Publishing.

Chapter 4

Hanson, R. (2009). *Buddha's Brain: The Practical Neuroscience of Happiness, Love, and Wisdom*. Oakland. New Harbinger Publications.

Singer, M. (2007). *The untethered soul: The journey beyond yourself*. Oakland. New Harbinger Publications.

Mental Health First Aid: https://www.mentalhealthfirstaid.org/author/rubinakapil/

Satchidananda, Sri Swami (1978). *The Yoga Sutras of Patanjali: Translation and Commentary*. Buckingham VA. Integral Yoga.

Chapter 5

Fritchen, J. (2016). Acute Metabolic Effects of Bulletproof Coffee (Doctoral dissertation).

Gruber, K. (2008). The Physiological and Psychological Effects of Ashtanga Yoga (Doctoral dissertation).

Hof, W. (2020). *The Wim Hof Method: Activate Your Potential, Transcend Your Limits*. London. Ebury Publishing.

Keng, S. L., Looi, P. S., Tan, E. L. Y., Yim, O. S., San Lai, P., Chew, S. H., & Ebstein, R. P. (2020). "Effects of Mindfulness-Based Stress Reduction on Psychological Symptoms and Telomere Length: A Randomized Active-Controlled Trial." *Behaviour Therapy* 51(6), 984-996.

Kerr, J. (2013). *Legacy*. London. Hachette UK.

Mujoriya, R., & Bodla, R. B. (2011). "A Study on Wheat Grass and its Nutritional Value." *Food Science and Quality Management* 2, 1-8. Random House.

Chapter 6

Frothingham, S. (2019). "How Long Does It Take or a New Behaviour to Become Automatic?"https://www.healthline.com/health/how-long-does-it-take-to-form-ahabit#the-21-day-myth

Hall, D., James, D., & Marsden, N. (2012). "Marginal Gains: Olympic Lessons in High Performance for Organisations." *HR Bulletin: Research and Practice* 7(2), 9-13.

Hardy, D. (2011). *The Compound Effect*. Boston. Da Capo Press.

Maurer, R. (2019). *The Spirit of Kaizen: Creating Lasting Excellence One Small Step at a Time*. New York. McGraw Hill.

Chapter 8

Bjork, E. L., & Bjork, R. A. (2011). "Making Things Hard on Yourself, but in a Good Way: Creating Desirable Difficulties to Enhance Learning." Psychology and the Real World: Essays Illustrating Fundamental Contributions to Society, 2(59-68).

Stern, E. (2019). One Simple Thing: A New Look at the Science of Yoga and How It Can Transform Your Life. New York. North Point Press.

PART II

Allen, D. (2015). *Getting Things Done: The Art of Stress-Free Productivity*. London. Penguin.

Banayan, A. (2018). *The Third Door: The Wild Quest to Uncover How the World's Most Successful People Launched Their Careers*. New York. Currency.

Bishop, J. (2010). *Faith*. https://plato.stanford.edu/entries/faith/. *Stanford Encyclopedia of Philosophy*.

Bjork, E. L., & Bjork, R. A. (2011). "Making Things Hard on Yourself, but in a Good Way: Creating Desirable Difficulties to Enhance Learning." *Psychology and the Real World: Essays Illustrating Fundamental Contributions to Society* 2(59-68).

Chokoisky, S. (2014). *The 5 Dharma Types. Ancient Wisdom for Discovering Your Purpose and Destiny*. New York. Simon and Schuster.

Coelho, P. (2014). *The Alchemist*. Glasgow. Singel Uitgeverijen.

Duckworth, A. (2017). *Grit: Why Passion and Resilience are the Secrets to Success*. London. Penguin Random House.

Dweck, C. (2017). *Mindset: Changing the Way You Think to Fulfil Your Potential*. New York. Hachette UK.

Eger, E. E. (2017). *The Choice: Even in hell Hope can Flower*. London. Penguin Random House.

Frankl, V. E. (1985). *Man's Search for Meaning*. Boston. Simon and

Schuster.

Gillihan, S. J. (2016). *Retrain Your Brain: Cognitive Behavioural Therapy in 7 Weeks: A Workbook for Managing Anxiety and Depression.* California. Althea Press.

Hambrick, D. Z., Oswald, F. L., Altmann, E. M., Meinz, E. J., Gobet, F., & Campitelli, G. (2014). "Deliberate practice: Is that all it takes to become an expert?" Intelligence, 45, 34-45.

Hill, N. (2011). *Think and Grow Rich, 71st Edition.* London. www. ThinkAndGrowRichGifts.com.au

Kishimi, I., & Koga, F. (2018). *The Courage to be Disliked: How to Free Yourself, Change Your Life and Achieve Real Happiness.* Crows Nest NSW. Atlantic Books.

Müller, E., Pröller, P., Ferreira-Briza, F., Aglas, L., & Stöggl, T. (2019). "Effectiveness of Grounded Sleeping on Recovery after Intensive Eccentric Muscle Loading. *Frontiers in Physiology* 10, 35.

Pychyl, T. A. (2013). *Solving the Procrastination Puzzle: A Concise Guide to Strategies for Change.* Tarcher Perigee.

Willink, J. (2017). *Discipline Equals Freedom: Field Manual.* New York. St. Martin's Press.

www.ingramcontent.com/pod-product-compliance
Lightning Source LLC
Chambersburg PA
CBHW061743270326
41928CB00011B/2351